BODY SENSE

BALANCING YOUR WEIGHT AND EMOTIONS

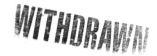
BODY SENSE

Balancing your weight and emotions

BRENDA CRAWFORD-CLARK

BEYOND
WORDS
Publishing
I N C

Beyond Words Publishing, Inc.
20827 NW Cornell Road, Suite 500
Hillsboro, Oregon 97124-9808
503-531-8700
1-800-284-9673

Design: Dorral Lukas and Principia Graphica
Composition: William H. Brunson Typography Services
Managing editor: Julie Steigerwaldt
Editor: Laura Carlsmith
Proofreaders: Carol Franks and Susan Beal

Printed in the United States of America
Distributed to the book trade by Publishers Group West

Library of Congress Cataloging-in-Publication Data

Crawford-Clark, Brenda.
    Body sense : balancing your weight and emotions / Brenda Crawford-Clark.
        p. cm.
    ISBN 1-58270-037-0 (pbk.)
        1. Compulsive eating.   2. Weight loss—Psychological aspects.
    3. Obesity—Psychological aspects.   4. Food habits.   I. Title.
    RC552.C65 C73   2001
    616.85'26—dc21

                                                                00-068079

The corporate mission of Beyond Words Publishing, Inc.:
    Inspire to Integrity

DEDICATION

To my husband Bob, whose unrelenting
encouragement and love has been my sustaining force
and
To my parents, who instilled in me a belief
that I could be who I want to be

contents

acknowLeDGmenTs

*No one goes his way alone; what we put
into the lives of others comes back into our own.*

—Anonymous

Humanity gets such a bad rap. I hope, as you read my acknowledge-ments, that although you do not know these generous people, their kindness will serve as a reminder that people are basically good and want to help each other.

Words of thanks seem like such a small recognition to the many people who have played a part in making my dream of publishing this book become a reality. However, know that behind the words are my heartfelt gratitude and appreciation. My life has been changed, as I hope yours will be, by all the people who opened their souls to me as together we explored their life connections. Their experiences and their willingness to search for answers are wonderful examples of strength and hope, and their lives have provided the inspiration for the stories you will read and the exercises you will work. I want to especially thank Karen, who not only shared her struggles and suc-cess, but asked that her name not be masked with a pseudonym, another step that allows her to break free of the past without shame and to accept her own wonderful transformation with pride. That step took a great deal of strength and courage, which she always had, but she didn't always know how to direct it to meet her goals. She's a wonderful person.

I am also indebted to the Maui Writer's Conference, which provided me with an opportunity to connect with Cynthia Black, the owner of Beyond Words Publishing, and Laura Carlsmith, the acquisitions editor, who helped nurture *Body Sense* to its publication. Equally important is my thanks to my husband, Bob, who has provided me unending encouragement; to my son, Matthew, who along with his staff at Kaleidoscope Enterprises turned my computer crises into learning experiences, and also to my daughter, Laura, whose sense of humor and willingness to take on menial tasks helped me maintain a balance during the writing of *Body Sense*. And, of course, there are other people along the way who have no idea they have influenced this book, including Bob Greene and Oprah Winfrey, whose excellent book *Make the Connection* prompted me to expand the focus of *Body Sense* because all who struggle with their weight share common issues.

And finally, my thanks are to God, who has been a partner in this endeavor from the beginning. Truly, no one does go his way alone.

Brenda

┤ INTRODUCTION ├

LIGHTEN YOUR SOUL, LIGHTEN YOUR BODY

Start by doing what's necessary, then what's possible;
And suddenly you are doing the impossible.

—St. Francis of Assisi

What Is Frustrating You?

Is it difficult for you to keep off lost weight, no matter what you do? Are you tired of clothes that don't fit? Are you frustrated at spending money on diets that don't work? Do you think of bathing suit season with anxiety? Are you sick of not eating what you want because of calories, fat, or guilt? Does your heart sink when your spouse says your weight is making you unattractive? Are you tired of feeling as if other people are judging what you eat? Do you want to explode if you hear one more kind soul giving you weight loss advice? Do you eat for emotional nourishment? Does concern about your weight take up a lot of your energy?

Have you suspected there is more to weight loss than just diets? Well, you're right.

In this book, you're going to learn how to make your weight problems go away, but it won't include traditional crazy diets, miracle cures, and more broken promises. It will include a strategic, body-sensible approach that is packed with information, new tools, and important life connections. You'll be asked to provide a little emotional sweat, but you'll realize an immediate payoff in everyday life. Quite honestly, before you shed the pounds, you will first begin to lose the emotional garbage, the key to sustained weight loss or weight stability. Any other approach is a prescription for futility.

Uncovering Hidden Connections

Have you ever considered the emotional issues that continue to strike back when you are focused on a new diet or exercise plan, working to lose weight? Emotions often drive people to use food—from a need for comfort or reward or as a way to rebel, stuff anger, or gain power or control.

It may surprise you to learn that many life events, such as the death of a loved one, loss of a career, miscarriage, divorce, incapacity due to an accident or illness, abuse, or lost dreams, can give birth to weight problems. In *Body Sense*, you'll learn what to do to counter the lingering effects on your emotions of past pain, trauma, and losses.

You'll also learn how to identify your feelings as messengers and how to take proactive steps to decrease your stress, frustration, and unhappiness. When you toss the emotional weight, you'll find the physical pounds will no longer be such a concern. You'll be more inclined to incorporate exercise into your daily life as a way to keep your total body healthy because you want to, not just as a drudging way to zap calories.

You may also be surprised to learn how your body's chemical reactions affect your weight. You'll discover that whether you choose to work out at the health club or to spend an afternoon playing cards with friends, both put into play chemical reactions that are strong appetite regulators and reduce your stress, which can contribute to weight loss.

Finally, after reading this book you'll have resources to examine the pieces of your unique life puzzle and make empowering changes. *Body Sense* will give you details of where to look for the hidden puzzle pieces, the parts of your life that you probably never realized could influence your eating and weight. Some of those pieces include the following:

- How residue from long-ago trauma interferes with your self-image, flooding you with feelings that drive you to use food.
- How loss that you thought you had dealt with can have a lingering effect on your life, resulting in your eating or missing meals to cope with the emotional aftereffects.
- How food has been meeting specific emotional needs and how you can learn powerful, more effective replacements.
- How years of negative self talk prevent you from having energy to make yourself a priority, thereby reinforcing unhealthful patterns of using food.
- How emotional, physical, or sexual trauma can create feelings flashbacks that pull you toward food for control and comfort.
- How family relationships and misperceptions are often connected to the use of food as a coping mechanism or as a means to reduce anger, rebel, or gain control and power.
- How an unresolved emotional issue can keep you stuck, unable to lose any more pounds once you reach a certain weight.
- How chemicals within your body are directly tied to how you feel about yourself and can affect your desire to use food.
- How hypoglycemia and food allergies can contribute to your using and reacting to certain foods.
- How a fear of conflict can keep you from setting boundaries to protect yourself.
- How confusion between rage and anger can keep you from using assertiveness and can push you to turn to food instead of expressing your needs.

As you can see, there are numerous factors that can contribute to weight problems, many of which you probably had no idea were connected to unwanted pounds. With that knowledge as ammunition, you're going to be progressing through *Body Sense*, analyzing how these different life components may have affected you, and gaining the specific tools you need not only to maintain a healthy long-term weight, but also provide you with emotional energy.

From Emotional Eating to Emotional Balance

In *Body Sense*, I'll share with you the process that I've developed during the past fifteen years as a director and therapist for hospital and outpatient programs specializing in eating disorders, trauma, substance abuse, and depression. It's a process that will steadfastly decrease the focus of weight in your life and replace emotional eating with emotional balance and a strong sense of a self, not dependent upon the scales. The process includes using the experiences of others to inspire hope and pull you out of the sense of isolation and failure that often builds with chronic weight problems. The exercises in the process have helped hundreds and will help you build a powerful base of self-knowledge and self-esteem.

I will share with you the same techniques that I have used successfully in my private practice, just as if you were sitting across from me. You'll learn why you have difficulties with food and your weight and how to gain control. You'll learn how to replace negative thoughts about yourself with a new belief system built upon the power of new information, acceptance, recognized strength, and hope for who you can be.

You'll also learn Ten Steps to Freedom, crucial actions in decreasing the importance of weight in your life. These steps also will help you identify your own progress as you let go of what has been holding you back.

You'll notice quotations at the beginning of each chapter and affirmations at the conclusion. These are additional tools to help you get quiet with yourself and learn to give yourself ongoing encouragement. Without an investment of your time and an acceptance of your self, weight loss will never be sustained. You'll find that, as you become more self-loving and make these important life connections, weight becomes less important. As this change occurs and you treat yourself well, one of two things usually happens: either you will continue to lose to a more healthy, comfortable weight, or you will stop the process of losing and then gaining more after each diet attempt.

About 80 percent of the people who actively engage in this process of change lose weight. Of course, you won't get that feel-good surge that you get from losing the first five pounds of water weight. A body-sensible loss is gradual, but it is sustainable. If you reach a plateau but are still not at a healthy weight, that's okay. You just need a little more work in this process. When you are ready to go ahead, it's your call. You can review previously read chapters and rework exercises to help you identify why there remains a temporary roadblock to continued weight loss. Regardless, you have discovered there is no need for drastic, restrictive diets, because you can now recognize when you are feeling over the edge, and you have the tools to pull yourself back and to take care of yourself in healthful ways. The scales may go up and down slightly, but ultimately you will have stopped the gaining trend.

Unfortunately, there will be that 20 percent who will still continue to hurt themselves with unreasonable diet regimens because they give little consideration to how they will feel six months down the road when the weight returns. If you find yourself leaning in that direction, remember the past. It can be difficult to have faith that there is anything to stop the cycle of yo-yo diets. But, if you follow the body-sense process, you'll find positive results.

Long-Term Changes

As you read and work through this book, you'll be making such a dramatic shift in how you think about yourself that your weight will no longer dictate who you are. You'll see yourself as a whole person, a spiritual being no longer restricted by your past perceptions. You'll be free to be whoever you want to be. You'll no longer define success in pounds but in loving, respecting, and encouraging yourself and others.

My hope is that you will see yourself in the stories, commit the time to complete the exercises, and incorporate what you learn into your everyday life.

Change is in your hands. But change won't occur if you just read the material in this book without doing the exercises. You need the exercises to pull together your thinking and your heart, the two key components in changing long-held, self-defeating beliefs and addressing problems successfully.

As you begin by sharing the stories of Karen and others in the first chapter, you will see that people who struggle with their weight have had experiences and feelings similar to yours. By reading about others who have won the battle against weight and, more importantly, felt more confident and secure within themselves, you can throw away the isolating or shame-filled thoughts of being a failure or different. You are not alone!

AFFIrmation
I am taking steps today to reach my full potential.

---- **1** ----

CHALLENGING OLD BELIEFS AND MAKING NEW CONNECTIONS

Whatever you do or dream you can, begin it.
Boldness has genius and power and magic in it.
—Johann von Goethe

Would you like to start a bonfire and load it with every low-fat, no-carb, nothing-that-tastes-good diet that you have ever tried and then ignite it with all the empty promises to end your weight problems? Go ahead. You don't need them anymore.

Consider this: 167 million men and women in the United States are on a diet at any given moment. If that many people are trying a solution and it doesn't work, something's wrong with the so-called solution. Contrary to what proponents of expensive diet regimens say, these diets can't work long term, no matter how much willpower you have. Why? Because they are missing essential connections. Even scientists researching weight loss medication acknowledge they will never be able to guarantee the same results with human beings as with animals because the factor of emotions always comes into play.

Your solution, therefore, doesn't lie in the next magic pill or diet, but in your attaining a balance between weight and emotions.

You can attain this balance, but first you'll have to challenge the beliefs you've held about weight loss. Challenging such deeply held beliefs may not be easy. These beliefs have been reinforced by a multi-million dollar diet industry that bases its success on your failure. By convincing you that your past dieting efforts haven't worked because you either haven't tried their plan or haven't had the willpower to remain on it, you've been positioned for the next buy.

Yet look around. How many people do you know who have started these plans and sustained long-term weight loss? Probably not too many. Most gain back all their weight within six months to a year. You can't stop weight concerns with a diet and a simple dose of willpower any more than willpower alone would mend a broken leg. The advertisements make you think that almost everyone is success-ful, and set you up to feel isolated if you are not. But the majority of people are just like you. You need only to look around at the grocery store as you peruse the frozen food aisle, or look at others in any weight-loss program. You're connected to these others who struggle with their weight in ways you may never have imagined. Similarities go far beyond your concern about appearance. With the stories in this book, you'll find deeper connections to others, connections you can use to break free of your own weight concerns.

Your challenge today is to put aside old beliefs and look at weight issues differently. Instead of assuming something is wrong with you, assume you have not had a complete package of information. With this book, you'll not only discover ways to lose weight, but you'll also rediscover yourself. You'll discover areas where you simply were stumped and could not go forward, because there were hidden emo-tional or physical factors hampering you.

For your own sake, resist the instinct to sneak peeks at the chapters ahead, because what you learn in one chapter prepares you for the next. You're doing more than just reading another diet book now. You've started a process, much like you would in an individual consultation. The stories will provide you with information you'll use to assess your own unique experiences. The exercises are oppor-tunities to learn more about yourself and, ultimately, to gain free-dom not only from diets but from any emotional and physical restraints that have held you back in your relationships, career, and enjoyment of life.

Connecting to the Source of It All

Your weight can be anchored to situations that you thought that you had dealt with. While you may have moved beyond them because of your own inner strengths, determination, and tendency to put the needs of others before your own, lingering emotions can remain repressed and make you vulnerable to their eruption later. And at that later time, you unfortunately have no connection to when or why they first occurred and are, therefore, less able to do anything about them. That's the scenario that pulls you back to food, no matter how determined you are to stick to a new diet.

Weight problems have a starting place, and going back to that place can help you end them. Often the seeds for weight problems are planted in childhood and grow gradually over the years. These can arise from misperceptions. You may have grown up feeling that you never met your parents' expectations or that you were smothered by their absorption and control in your life, however well intentioned. As one young woman described her relationship, "I didn't know where my mother ended and I began." Or, you may have suffered at the other end of that spectrum, in a home where parents were either absent because of divorce or work, or were physically present but emotionally unavailable.

If you came from an alcoholic or abusive home, your risk of having weight problems is higher because, in emotionally chaotic homes, there may be a strong tendency to mask problems and not own feelings. Eating or not eating could help you distance yourself from the hurt. Growing up, you may have been expected to assume adult roles. You may never have had the chance to be a child. You may have been "the man of the house" or even a surrogate spouse or parent. If you were a child expected to perform in an adult world, you skipped important developmental stages. Typically, children do not function well when they attempt to fill an adult role, and they can suffer emotional harm that follows them into adulthood.

Society can create stress and loss if you were a child who initially was even only a little overweight. Children often ridicule and ostracize the overweight child. Parents, attempting to protect the child, may exert a lot of pressure to lose weight. It does not matter if you are 102 pounds overweight or one. Feeling pressured about weight distorts how you look at your body, setting you up to feel insecure and unhappy.

In the pages that follow, you'll uncover your own starting point and ways to reclaim your life. Whatever the origins of your weight problems, sharing the experiences of others will touch your heart and remind you of the power of strength, of hope, and, most important, of work focused on the emotional causes of weight problems.

Sharing Strengths and Hope

Lucy, a successful career woman, began turning to food to fill the gaping hole in her heart when her mother died. Though her family attempted to fill the void, the ten-year-old's life would never be the same. Never again could she pick up the telephone and call Mom when she needed her, never again listen to her laughter, play crazy games with her, or confide important secrets. Relationships in her family also changed. Her father's grief and the stress of being a single parent took him away. The emptiness and loneliness were immense, and Lucy tried to fill them with food. As she grew older, she also turned to people with the same expectation: that they could take away the loneliness and fill the void left when her mother died. She fell into a pattern of negative relationships with men who appeared emotionally available on the surface but who actually had little to give. She lost herself in jobs that gave her nothing in return, yet she stayed out of a feeling of loyalty and a drive to try harder. The loyalty gave her a false sense of closeness, a feeling she had longed for since her mother died. Lucy increasingly relied on food for solace, with no idea that the answer to her weight problems lay in uncovering their origin. Instead, she tried one diet after another, unsuccessfully, until she realized she had to take the first step in shaking the old albatross: challenging her beliefs, the first of ten steps to freedom.

Ten Steps to Freedom

1. Challenge your old beliefs about yourself, your weight, and problem solving.
2. Take charge to get your past off your plate.
3. Burn your negative self-talk garbage.
4. Identify your feelings and analyze their purpose; then take appropriate actions to care for yourself.
5. Learn where to get control—and when to let it go.
6. Own, and then let go of your losses.
7. Make anger work for you: Identify how your ideas about anger and rage were shaped by your environment growing up, and learn more effective ways to express yourself today.
8. Recognize the presence of chemical reactions that affect your weight.
9. Choose a strategic plan of eating that meets your unique needs and lifestyle.
10. Review your progress, take note of your changes, and celebrate yourself!

Each of these steps is described in detail in chapters 3 through 11.

Step 1: Challenge your old beliefs about yourself, your weight, and problem solving.

You have not failed because you haven't tried hard enough. Acknowledge the emotional factor in your weight issues. Acknowledge that you are not alone, that you have similarities with others that go beyond the scales. By increasing your understanding of yourself and connections to life events, you can end your weight struggles and increase your self-acceptance.

Challenging what you've been taught to believe is probably the most crucial step of all. It removes you from the sense of shame, failure, and isolation that the diet industry has put upon you. It puts you in a position for learning and for openness to change. It gives you the base for progressing through the next nine steps, the steps that will make a difference not only in your weight but also in improving your energy, self-confidence, and focus.

Lucy related, "When I realized that my eating problems began when I lost my mom, it made sense to me why I couldn't shake my weight with a diet. I had started eating for a reason, and that reason could never be met with food. I could never replace my mother. Once I realized that, I took myself out of the diet frenzy and began concentrating on the other steps that helped me learn better ways to meet my needs."

You'll have the opportunity to process through each of the same steps as Lucy, with detailed instructions and guidance throughout each chapter. As you can see, none of these steps are insurmountable. Tackling your weight problems is a very doable task. It just means you are going to have to make yourself your project as you advance through these steps.

As Lucy progressed through the steps, she said, "I found myself gradually feeling better with each step. I didn't give up food. I found I didn't have to. I didn't have to be perfect on a strict diet; I was able to put the stress out of my eating. As I did, little by little, the pounds started to come off. Now, my weight varies in a five-pound range.

"I know I sometimes eat more than I should, but I don't get bent out of shape about it. I've learned to step back and look at whether I'm eating because of a physical or emotional hunger, and I now know actions to take if it's not physical. That's all I have to do. I don't have to jump into some diet that is going to make me miserable for the next three months, and then miserable again three months after I stop it because I start gaining the weight back."

Jack, a forty-seven-year-old carpenter, had a similar transition as he progressed through the steps and learned more about himself. His problems with his weight began not in childhood but after an event later in life. Jack injured himself in a fall and was unable to return to the same type of work. For months he struggled with pain, unemployment, and the stress of looking for a new career. Food became his best friend, as he ate to push down the fear, anger, and guilt that came from not being able to support his family. Food altered his emotions momentarily, but instead of feeling better about himself, he gained fifty-five pounds and felt much worse. With his doctor's help, he tried medically supervised diets, yet Jack couldn't shake the emotions that kept driving him toward food and away from physical activity. Jack related, "I had to allow myself to consider that my weight problems began with the fall and that maybe I hadn't dealt with my emotions as well as I thought. That's pretty tough for a man. I didn't even like admitting I had these emotions. I was worried I would seem weak. But when I allowed for that possibility and began working those steps of analyzing the emotions, then accepting that they served a purpose, and then finding out how to act upon them, I gradually saw my eating habits change. I began to realize when I was eating for an emotion, and had learned other ways to take care of that emotion. The binges had only made me feel worse, ultimately. Now, I've been steadily losing those extra pounds, and I feel like getting out with the kids and just enjoying myself."

Maggie's eating problems originated to stave off the same emotions as Jack's, but her feelings were anchored to her husband's telling her he wanted a divorce. She was filled with fear of being alone and supporting herself, with extreme guilt because she mistakenly agreed with her husband that she alone was to blame, and with anger at him and at herself. She felt as if her life was out of control. Similar feelings, different causes than Jack's and Lucy's, yet they triggered the same difficulties with eating. Maggie alternated between periods of not eating at all and eating small amounts of food nonstop. This cycle continued long after the divorce was final. She said, "I know now that I ate because I felt so out of control, and owning or acting upon any of those other feelings frightened me, especially anger. Since then, I've learned that I have to honor those feelings and that I have so many choices about what kind of actions I can take. I stopped that up-and-down eating, and that stopped my weight gain."

As you continue to share the experiences of others, consider whether you are using eating to change your emotions.

Using Food for Control

Like Maggie, the more out of control your life feels, the more you may rely on food to attempt to gain control or comfort. It can start with not eating parts of a meal, then gradually missing meals. Or, eating cookies when you feel intense loneliness or stress, and then gradually relying on more and more food. Each experience of this numbing-by-food takes you farther away from recognizing where the emotional pain originated. Gradually, using food becomes an automatic, immediate reaction. Pain triggers a craving for food or some other eating behavior. As energy becomes focused on meeting that need, you lose touch with the source of the pain and with any chance of effectively decreasing it. In the chapters that follow, you'll learn how to interrupt this process, just as Lucy, Jack, and Maggie did.

Perhaps you also will connect with Karen's experiences. Although Karen's weight conflict progressed into an eating disorder before she got help, the bottom-line issues remain the same. While the other anecdotes in this book are composites of many with weight concerns, Karen asked to tell her own story. She is no longer ashamed of who she is.

Karen, thirty-six, is both an incest survivor and in recovery for bulimia and anorexia. It was not unusual for her to binge when she was feeling bad and then to purge by downing up to twenty laxatives at a time. She suffered through numerous negative relationships and three destructive marriages, always lost, feeling incompetent and incapable every day of her life. Here's her story:

"I could not even go out to eat without being afraid people would make fun of me because of my weight. I let the scales tell me how to feel. I let my ex-husband dictate who my friends were and what I did. I was afraid to stand up for myself and tell him how I felt, for fear I would lose him and be all alone."

Her struggles and recovery have been intense, yet healing. Her persistence and hope have led her to important catalysts in ending her long-term weight struggles and in changing her life. The most dramatic change occurred when she began practicing Step 2 (getting your past off your plate) and was able to stop overwhelming feelings from the past intruding on her life. In doing that, she immediately felt more in control and, therefore, more self-confident, a mindset that gave her the potential to look more clearly at situations. Using the same tools you'll learn about in chapter 3, Karen began to shrug off the claim the past had on her. She gained control of her emotions, thoughts and reactions, control that then eliminated her need to use her eating disorder to hide or express emotions. She concluded, "When I look back, I have always used food as a friend. Since I was a little child, when my mother and father were fighting, I would head for the kitchen. For the first time, I have learned to let myself feel without numbing out by reaching for food. In doing so, I am exorcising myself of a lot of guilt which I have learned I did not deserve. I am setting boundaries. It finally makes sense why diets never worked."

It also was difficult for Karen to realize that her caretaking personality, where she consistently put others' needs before her own, did not pay off in people loving or caring for her more. When she completed Steps 3 (burning your self-talk garbage) and 4 (caring for yourself) and began routinely setting boundaries, she discovered that people who didn't honor those boundaries had been draining her energy and emotions with their needs, but they were giving little other than words in return. Karen finally realized why she felt alone. With that difficult recognition, she made the choice to discontinue some relationships, creating more space for healthier friendships with people who were respectful of her as a person. She also found herself re-examining boundaries; she learned that saying "no" paid off at her job, where she had been working too many hours for her pay. She asked for and received a raise, and she established clear boundaries for the time she would be available for work. She was then able to explore new career opportunities with the time and energy she had freed.

Karen began to ask herself questions: "Sometimes I asked myself, 'What am I doing all this emotional work for?' There were times I dredged up things that seemed just too painful to bear. Then I was reminded I have always carried that pain. The difference was, by laying it out on the table, I was finally able to tap into the solutions that others had used to work through similar experiences and let the pain go.

"I learned it all comes down to feeling the feelings that the little girl and the adult she grew into had stuffed for all those years. I can break that old behavior and develop new and healthy behaviors by slowing down and finding out what I am feeling, whether it takes ten minutes or half an hour.

"I am not the same person today. In change, we develop inner strength. We become capable. We become ourselves. We need to do the work necessary. We need to feel the pain. Validate it and do something with it. We need to let the emotions come through us and not stuff them down with eating, drinking, sex—whatever your drug of choice may be—because it doesn't work. We would just continue with that miserable life.

"I remember there were many times I couldn't imagine being any different. It is gradual. You just plug away. You do what you need to do—and see the changes. Then you find yourself saying. Oh my God. I CAN do this!

"For the first time in my life, I feel I have choices. I am alive. I have hope. Today I have a tomorrow."

Solutions, Not Diets

As you shared the experiences of others, did you consider how many of their weight issues could have been solved by a diet? None, not a one.

Lucy, Jack, Maggie, and Karen learned that the solutions they had been chasing were only empty promises and that, until they challenged their old beliefs, their weightier problems remained. The steps they talked about are the ones you will progress through in the following chapters. Years of experience have been translated into a very effective process. It's not mystical. It only requires attention to you, given by the person who probably gives you the least—yourself.

Now that you've successfully challenged old beliefs and freed yourself from the guilty thinking that kept you moving from one diet to another, you're ready to continue your progression by adding insight and tools to make long-lasting changes. In the chapters ahead, you'll progress through the next nine steps that will aid you in this journey. In addition to building new skills, each step will reinforce what you have already learned in previous chapters. In chapter 2, you'll complete two questionnaires that will help you to begin to uncover patterns and reasons for your use of food, examining the difference between stress eating and compulsive overeating. Soon, you'll reach the point where you are so comfortable about what you have learned that you will no longer have to be as conscientious about using your newfound knowledge because it will become a natural part of who you are. As you relate to the stories and look through eyes of others, you'll learn new ways to gain compassion for yourself and encourage yourself while reinforcing your strengths.

Weight loss was never about willpower at all. The key has always been getting to know yourself.

AFFIrmation
Today I'm opening new doors
by challenging beliefs that kept me trapped.

2

TWENTY QUESTIONS (AND THEN SOME MORE)

. . . No one who learns to know himself
remains just what he was before.

—Thomas Mann

Before we move on to Step 2, getting your past off your plate, it's time for a little soul-searching. The questions that follow will help explain why diets do not, and cannot, work for everyone. If you answer yes to many of these questions, you are relying too much on food to medicate or replace uncomfortable feelings. Of course, everyone reaches for food at times to satisfy some unquenched need, whether it is eating potato chips on the way to a job interview or piling more on our plate after a stressful day at work. However, you can gradually reach a point where certain stresses occur and you automatically reach for food instead of identifying your needs and problem-solving them. As a result, both your emotional and physical needs are neglected.

With the tools and information you're gaining as you progress through the next nine chapters, you'll be able to identify how to meet those needs much more effectively, and therefore reduce your emotional need for food.

Stress Eating

Stress eating is using food to change your current emotional state. You may use it to reduce anxiety, fear, or depression. You may also eat when you are overwhelmed, need to reward yourself, need to gain more power or control, rebel, or push down anger. Food is used as an emotional replacement during stress eating, although its effects are only temporary.

You're not alone if you're turning to food when you're under stress; stress is a major contributor to weight gain in our society. As you answer the following questions, begin to expand your ideas of when and why you eat. When you recognize a connection between stress and eating, you can break that pattern by using the alternatives you'll learn later in the book.

When and Why You Eat

1. If you monitored your eating, would it increase substantially during times of stress?
2. Do you have a high degree of stress or chronic stress in your life?
3. Do you find it difficult to stop eating after you start?
4. Do you know what feelings drive you to eat?
5. Do you eat when you feel things are out of control?
6. Do you eat when you are anxious?
7. Do you eat when you are sad or depressed?
8. Do you eat as a reward?
9. Are you able to identify these feelings as they occur, prior to eating?
10. Have you tried to do something besides eat at that time?
11. Do you ever use food as a way to numb out or to avoid something painful?
12. Do you find yourself unhappy about your weight, but not doing anything about it?
13. Have you tried diets?
14. Do you find yourself eating fast?
15. Have you used food to get you through a difficult time?
16. Does your weight affect your self-esteem?
17. Do you have mood swings?
18. Do you ever use food to alter your mood?

19. Do you "forget to eat" and miss meals when you are under stress?
20. Do you overeat?
21. Do you eat when you are bored?
22. Do you eat when you are frustrated?
23. Do you eat when you feel inadequate?
24. Do other people focus on your weight?
25. Do you notice that you are craving or eating the same food during emotional times?

Congratulations! You have taken an important step in discovering how and why you use food. As you learn to rely less on food for stability, your weight will become less of a problem.

Compulsive Overeating

If you continue to rely on food to mask or handle your emotions, stress eating can develop into compulsive overeating. This type of eating usually causes greater weight gain and frequently interferes in other areas of your life because food becomes a primary focus.

Compulsive overeating includes all the components of stress eating, but it is more driven. As it progresses, the eating feels more out of control. If you are a compulsive overeater, it is extremely difficult to limit the quantity of what you are eating. Instead of having one candy bar, you may have two or three. Instead of eating a piece of cake, you may eat several—or even the whole cake. As you advance further into compulsive overeating, you often will feel guilt, shame, and depression after the initial positive emotional payoff from eating wears away.

Answer the following questions to begin to identify patterns to your eating and to why you are aching for food.

1. Do you find yourself eating when you're not hungry?
2. Do you often eat alone?
3. Are you afraid to eat in public?

4. Have you tried numerous diets, only to lose weight and gain more back?
5. Do you have mood swings?
6. Do you live to eat rather than eat to live?
7. Do you have low self-esteem?
8. Are you irritable?
9. Are you unhappy or depressed?
10. Have you become isolated because you have eliminated social activities?
11. Are you frequently embarrassed?
12. Do you believe people are often looking at you and thinking or talking about your weight or appearance?
13. Do you binge or eat to relieve anxiety?
14. Do you find yourself being dishonest to cover your eating habits or to keep the peace at home?
15. Do you live to please other people?
16. Do you find yourself believing you never have time for yourself?
17. Do you feel guilty frequently, especially about eating?
18. Do you find it difficult to resist some foods?
19. Have you ever started thinking that you would eat just one cookie or favorite food, and then continued even when you were not hungry?
20. Do you ever plan a binge in advance?
21. Do you ever eat because you deserve a reward?
22. Do you find yourself either repressing your anger or holding it in until it explodes?
23. Or, do you feel angry all the time?
24. Are you a compulsive shopper?
25. Do you have frequent physical pains?
26. Do you believe your self-worth is dependent upon your losing weight?
27. Do you believe your weight causes problems in your relationships?

28. Is it difficult for you to ask for help?
29. Do you suffer from tiredness or apathy?
30. Do you ever feel emotionally numb?
31. Do you skip breakfast or lunch and then binge at night?
32. Do you have unreasonable resentments?
33. Is it difficult for you to discuss problems?
34. Do you become overwhelmed?
35. Do you have a preoccupation with eating or food?

If you answered yes to a significant number of these questions, you may be suffering from compulsive overeating, nonpurging bulimia, or depression associated with significant weight gain. That information is not meant to be overwhelming, only to allow you to understand why your past diet efforts don't signify that you have been a failure in any way. You just didn't have the complete package of information you needed to make internal changes that would be sustaining.

Pat yourself on the back again. It's not easy completing the questionnaires you have tackled, particularly if you have been laden with the feeling that something is wrong with you because you cannot control your weight and that it is a hopeless proposition to try to change. Get ready to throw those ideas out. With the knowledge you've already gained, you know there is no reason to feel shamed or incapable.

As you can see, your battle with weight goes beyond dieting. If you have answered yes to a significant number of the questions, you owe it to yourself to gather more information. Much of it is right in your hands. With information comes power and, finally, the true ability to change. For those of you who think your eating problems may have advanced into eating disorders such as anorexia and bulimia, see the additional questionnaires in the appendix. You'll also find help using these same tools and exercises.

In the next chapter, you'll learn about the often-overlooked effects of core feelings that are attached to past pain and about how to stop these feelings from triggering you into emotional eating. By learning how they began and how they can flood you with uncomfortable emotions today, you'll be gaining a crucial missing link in feeling better about your appearance. You have started the journey of learning how to be happy with who you are, no matter what the scales read.

AFFIRMATION
Today I look gently at myself
and embrace the journey
to discover who I am.

3

GET YOUR PAST OFF YOUR PLATE

And the day came when the risk it took to remain tight
inside the bud was more painful than the risk it took to blossom.

—Anaïs Nin

Imagine hanging up the telephone after a friend calls to break your date. Your heart sinks. Feelings of intense loneliness and rejection wash over you. You knock those away because they do not make sense. Within minutes, you find yourself craving something special from the kitchen. Food provides comfort. With each bite, you find yourself getting further from the intensity of the pain, dissociating with the powerful drug of food.

Later, you'll suffer from feelings of recrimination, anger, and maybe even disgust—not directed at your friend, but at yourself. Now food is no longer your best friend. It has become a powerful enemy that has tipped the scales against you. Whether you gain weight or not after emotional eating, your world is colored by distorted perceptions. You feel fat. It may seem harder to zip your jeans. Dressing for work may turn into a depressing, embarrassing scene as you fling one outfit after another on the bed because none of them seem to fit anymore. By the time you get to work, feelings of inadequacy begin slowly to envelop you. To the outside world, you look as if you have it all together. Inside, you are quivering. When your boss questions you about a project deadline, you despair: "She must not think I am doing this right. I must not be doing this right. *I can't do anything good enough.*"

Your mind turns to the candy bar you have hidden in your drawer. Chocolate would really taste good right now. In moments, the candy is gone. You are distanced from the despair, but a fog of uneasiness remains. When you see your boss again, your heart starts to race. Fear spikes, then dissipates as you replace it with thoughts of what you will get to eat on your way home. You may even consider which route to take in order to drive by just the right food establishments.

You are physically and emotionally exhausted by the time you begin your drive home. Now hours removed from the trigger that began this latest bout of emotional eating, you indulge yourself with special treats. Yes, the zipper was really tight after lunch, but you have switched into "What the heck, it doesn't matter anyway" mode. At this point, you may as well substitute "I" for "it." "*I don't matter anyway.*"

Something very complex happened here. You entered your unique Cycle of Pain that can spiral you downward from one negative reaction to the next. As you complete this chapter, you'll disassemble that Cycle piece by piece to take away its power. Given insight into its complexity, you'll understand how "Do Not Eat" notes on the refrigerator don't have a punch powerful enough to interrupt the cycle. You'll also better understand the reason you use food to change your emotions, and you will let go of more shame or guilt that you have held onto because of your weight.

You'll understand why losing yourself in the food didn't begin when you walked in the door after work. The cancellation by your friend triggered the first reaction. The question from the boss triggered the spiraling of a second reaction. But why the intensity? And, why the pattern of using food to get away from or to express feelings? How do you stop it?

Step 2: Take charge to get your past off your plate.
Sometimes emotions from the past resurface, particularly if in the past you have suffered trauma and loss. In the following pages, you'll be introduced to several new terms to help you understand how those

emotions contribute to your use of food. These definitions are also tools. They give you a way to define what is happening to you and will take away any sense that you are not normal, or that you are out of control, or that your battle with your weight is hopeless. Just using these words helps you remove yourself from past pain and get back into the present where you can take action. As we saw in chapter 1, stopping patterns of emotional eating is not as simple as managing calorie and fat count. It involves first exploring where your pain originated and how it affects you today, then examining patterns and, finally, changing the inappropriate actions that reinforce your own Cycle of Pain.

The Cycle of Pain

If you are troubled with emotional eating, you have events, thoughts, and experiences that trigger one another in a sequential cycle. Your use of food is only one part of that cycle. Understanding each component will help you interrupt reactions that quickly take you from an unbearable feeling into the destructive use of food.

Learning how each segment of the cycle relates to the others will give you tools to decrease stress and regain control quickly. You will be able to stop the cycle and experience new freedom and choices. You'll be able to use the energy that was being drained from you to explore some of the things you have always wanted to do. When you understand why you need to use food, you can meet that need in more healthful ways. The first step is understanding the process. Then you will learn how to change it.

It may be difficult initially to connect your emotions with your use of food. Over the years, using food to alter an emotion may have become an automatic response. This practiced disconnection removes you from the source of pain and prevents you from doing anything about it.

As you become more familiar with how some things trigger your use of food, you can take apart the Cycle of Pain. You may initially be surprised and even overwhelmed to discover how many occurrences are triggering you. But when you identify the feeling, you can begin to unravel the cause. For example, Tony, a forty-five-year-old man with chronic weight problems, was able to identify telephone calls with his mother as a trigger to his eating. The call triggered destructive messages of feeling not good enough. Triggering these perceptions may or may not have been his mother's intent, yet they were overwhelming. He would hang up the telephone and feel terrible. Tony recalled, "I would turn to my wife and just be shaking. I'd leave the room without saying a word, go off by myself, and flip on the television. This feeling of shame was just enveloping me. Something's wrong with me. It wasn't long before I'd find myself in the kitchen cooking a massive meal. The food was going to take me away from that feeling and the overbearing thought that, if my own mother thought this about me, I must be really bad.

"Of course, I was really disconnected from giving a name to those feelings. My body just kicked into survival mode, and I headed for the kitchen. It was only after I learned to acknowledge those feelings that I realized I had always carried them around. They interfered at work and at home. Food was something I used to help ease the load. And failed diets just reinforced the feelings and message I was running from.

"By identifying how I let one thing trigger another in my Cycle of Pain, I was able to interrupt that automatic progression from a feeling to food. I learned I did not have to feel that way. With lots of practice and shaky moments, I learned how to set boundaries with my mother and force a clarification of what was being said—the messages under the messages. When I did that, I gave myself permission to listen to my feelings and then take action based on their purpose.

"It didn't happen overnight, and it took a lot of work. But the result is I no longer seek food as my savior. And, after some initial struggles, I have a much better relationship with my mother than ever before. Most important, I'm starting to shake off the power of that feeling in directing my life in so many other areas. Because I felt something was wrong with me, I was letting people take advantage of me, and I stayed stuck in a job I didn't like because I was afraid I wasn't good enough to get another decent job.

"Before I could do anything about my pain, I had to acknowledge I was in it. That was scary to me, because I had spent a lifetime running from those feelings. But once I faced them, I didn't spend any more time numbing out over a plateful of my favorite food. Today I eat when I want to, not because an emotion is telling me to take care of it with food."

You'll find, too, that while at times it may be uncomfortable and even scary breaking through your own unique Cycle of Pain, you'll be rewarded with such a sense of relief and freedom that you'll be willing to keep moving through and even look forward to completing the work you'll begin in the next section.

Triggers to the Cycle of Pain

The Cycle of Pain is activated by a trigger, which may be a feeling, event, or misperception. As you can see in the following diagram, the trigger is quickly followed by feelings flashbacks, then by core feelings that activate core messages. These messages are so intense that you counter with defense reactions and then use some type of dissociation as a coping mechanism. That's the point in the cycle that you would use food self-destructively in an attempt to alter your mood. The food provides a brief respite, only to be followed by a negative feelings flashback about yourself, a flashback that again pushes you through the cycle.

For example, if you were abused as a child, you may overreact when a spouse questions a decision. Instead of reacting with an explanation, you may be flooded with core feelings of being judged, stupid, and not good enough. Those are often accompanied with a core message that automatically plays in your head, such as "I can't do anything right." You may react by withdrawing, not by problem solving. Afraid of a confrontation because of what you experienced as a child, you may resort to dissociating to get out of that fearful, angry mood. Yet, the feelings stay churning below the surface and can drive you to eat, purge, or binge to alter your mood. And unfortunately, the distance between you and your spouse grows.

Cycle of Pain

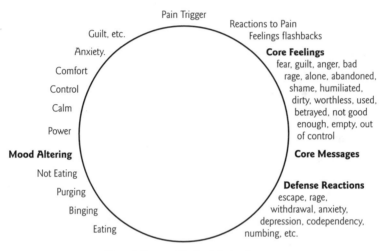

Dissociations as Coping Mechanism

Allow yourself to have an open mind as you consider how your past experiences have influenced your life. Don't hold back for fear this acknowledgement will label you a hopeless victim. On the contrary, if you have survived a traumatic experience, then by definition you have a wealth of inner resources. While acknowledging that you did suffer is difficult, denial never makes trauma go away. It only delays your actively doing something to put it to rest. Expand your view of trauma as you consider if it has influenced your life.

Traumas comes in all shapes and sizes, some less obvious than others. You may be like many people who believe they have "dealt with it and have gone on," thereby willing away any effects. Emotional, sexual, or physical abuse or crises leave trauma residues. Accidents, death, divorce, separation, and many other types of loss can also spark intense reactions. Threats of abandonment or verbal battering can tear one's heart apart and fill it with negative beliefs and messages. Repeated school failures can build into trauma. Lost dreams can be traumatic. In chapter 7, "Owning Your Hidden Losses," you'll learn more about what to do when loss is traumatic.

> **Trauma**
>
> *Trauma is any situation or event that causes you intense emotional or behavior disturbance. To understand the potential effect of a traumatic situation, we must look at it through your eyes when you experienced it. How old were you, and what supports did you have? What was happening in your life at the time? What type of environment were you in? What were the immediate effects? How did you cope with it?*

Trauma Bonds

Trauma bonds are an unpleasant trio in the Cycle of Pain, consisting of feelings flashbacks, core feelings, and core messages that pull you into past pain. Trauma bonds operate best when they remain unexamined. But they can be dismantled when you have knowledge of how they work and take direct action to stop their interference in your life.

It can be helpful to think of a trauma bond as similar to the large rope that holds a ship to the dock. The rope is made strong by the interweaving of several smaller threads. As you read and complete the exercises in the following chapters, think of yourself as having a small hacksaw in your hand and actively sawing through that trauma bond, piece by piece. Every bit of work you do helps tear it apart.

Muting core feelings by using food does not make pain go away. It simply pushes pain down into a holding spot. Core feelings—part of the trauma bond—remain inside and grow, dictating to and directing you as unseen messengers. These feelings have incredible power. Your core feelings can become a base for emotional development. They shape how you see yourself and can severely limit your potential. They can become part of your belief system.

Core Feelings

When you have been through a traumatic event or loss, you react with extremely strong feelings. Until you can voice these feelings, they remain a lasting connection to your pain.

In this list of core feelings, circle those that you recognize as having felt today before you used food. Next, if you recall a traumatic situation or loss from your past, draw a box around the feelings you felt at that time. Add any intense feelings you have had that you suspect are core feelings.

Abandoned	Fearful	Powerless
Alone	Guilt	Rejected
Bad	Hopeless	Stupid
Betrayed	Humiliated	Trapped
Defective	Not Good	Unlovable
Dirty	Enough	Unworthy
Empty	Out of Control	

As you can see on the Cycle of Pain diagram, core feelings inevitably trigger core messages. Born as coping mechanisms to get through a traumatic event or loss, core messages usually take the form of a destructive attack on yourself in which you either deny the traumatic situation took place or assume undeserved responsibility for it. It is crucial that you identify your unique core messages in the words that you use. Some examples are these: "I'm not any good if I don't lose weight." "I'm responsible if anything bad happens." "I can't do anything right." "I am a failure if I make a mistake." "Something must be wrong with me." Identifying these core messages strips them of their power over you. Acknowledging these feelings lessens their grip on you. You disable the connections to past trauma, you learn healthier responses, and you discover that your need for food decreases. Later in the book, you'll learn more ways to disrupt and destroy core messages.

The next important step is understanding the concept of feelings flashbacks and then beginning to control them, first by acknowledging when they are occurring.

Feelings flashbacks knock you back into a moment of extreme vulnerability and pain, although the trigger today may actually be harmless. Within a moment, your confidence fails and you feel frozen with fear, agitated to rage, or incredibly alone in the world—the same core feelings you experienced at the time of the initial trauma. You may not know this process is occurring because it happens within seconds. During feelings flashbacks, you may feel a knot in your stomach, your heart sink, or depression envelop you like a cloud. You may feel smothered, numb, or as if your heart is racing. Feelings flashbacks are usually followed by destructive self talk in the form of core messages that are tied to already existing self-doubts.

Unhealthy Defense Reactions

Reactions, or coping mechanisms, vary, but the ultimate goal is to get rid of those overwhelming feelings as quickly as possible. To cope with difficult situations, you may engage in defense reactions learned long ago. However these defense mechanisms began, as time passes from the initial event, they most often become destructive. They include escape, rage, withdrawal, anxiety, depression, and people-pleasing.

Dissociation

Sometimes we are so intent on getting through to a place where we can function that we don't honor our feelings during stressful times. Often, we don't even validate the pain. In cases of severe trauma, a life-saving technique is to dissociate from it. Dissociation begins as an automatic coping mechanism when a traumatic event occurs. It removes you from the physical and emotional pain of a situation either by going someplace else within your mind, blanking out to deny it is happening, numbing in order to escape feelings, or focusing intently on something else. Unfortunately, for many people, dissociation becomes a coping skill, as they learn to rely on self-destructive behaviors to dissociate from any stressful situation. But coping is not truly living.

Eating, bingeing, restricting food, and purging can all be used to dissociate or change your moods. They initially can bring feelings of power, calm, control, and comfort, but soon those feelings are replaced by core feelings of being anxious, guilty, and out of control. These negative feelings will trigger you back into the Cycle of Pain.

Stopping the Cycle

Throughout this book, you're going to learn more about attacking each segment of the Cycle of Pain. Think of your work as an attack, because attack is a powerful word that implies you are very much in charge and are taking needed action. To understand your unique cycle and your progress as you lessen its impact, draw your own circle diagram. Around the diagram, write the following headings: pain trigger, core feelings, core messages, defense reactions, dissociation coping mechanisms, and mood-altering action. Fill in the blanks with your reactions as you progress through *Body Sense* and identify what is pulling you down. These are all things you can change. For example, if you learn that "abandoned" is one of your core feelings, add it to your drawing to help you target it as you work in later chapters to express your feelings, to explore control, loss, and anger. Your notation will also be a reminder to watch for overreactions, which will signal the need for you to explore further why this feeling continues to erupt and what actions you need to take instead of progressing into the Cycle of Pain. If the core feeling is being triggered constantly, you will also want to examine current relationships to determine whether it is being reinforced by others in your environment.

When you take action to interrupt this cycle, draw a line through the core feeling, core message, defense reaction, or mood altering action that your work has attacked. Make a note of your new feeling, or action. It is not unusual to draw a line through the same reaction several times as you learn how far-reaching its effects have been and new ways to stop the pattern. Your Cycle of Pain will begin to fall apart to be replaced by a Cycle of Health. You will begin to shatter the automatic progression of self-sabotage. In this way, your drawing will provide a visual reminder of your power to make changes.

You'll learn to replace core feelings with increased confidence, and with feelings of being worthy, focused, and in control. Your defense reactions will be much more effective, as you learn to substitute effective conversation and self-care techniques. You'll accept feelings instead of discarding them. By accepting feelings, you will be more empowered to take effective actions. Best of all, you will no longer have to rely on food as a mood-altering ally.

Grounding Techniques

Grounding techniques will help you move out of emotional flooding by achieving a balance between thinking and feeling. These techniques are helpful in any stressful situation, but they are essential to break free of a trauma bond. Grounding techniques allow you to separate yourself from the emotion long enough to do something about it.

When you are overrun with emotions, do something concrete instead of reaching for food or getting lost in a spiral of feelings and the need to dissociate. Concrete actions mean making a choice. This action in itself helps break the emotional chain reaction. Choosing to stop and think, to write, to get up and move about puts you in charge.

Grounding techniques also put your feet solidly in the present and protect you from overreacting or feeling incapable of taking any action. It may sound simplistic, but doing the following affirmations is the first step in taking you out of a self-destructive cycle and anchoring you firmly in control.

Tell yourself the following: My name is _____. I am _____ years old. I am in a safe place. If I am not, I can leave. I can choose what I do next. (You may want to add your own personal anchors to reality, such as your address, job, and primary support people in your life.)

By identifying a situation or person as stressful, you have begun to take control. If you take it one step further and begin to identify what emotions you are feeling, you are further breaking the Cycle of Pain. By identifying emotions, you begin to take ownership and can then look at your choices. What is the purpose of the emotion? Am I overreacting? Is this person's actions or this situation making me feel this way? What do I need to do to change how I feel instead of using food? In chapters 4 and 5, you'll learn additional grounding techniques.

Annie's Story

You may be surprised by how frequently feelings flashbacks have been occurring and the amount of distortion they create in our lives. Annie, 46, struggled with her weight for years. She relates her experience:

"When I learned what feelings flashbacks are, I realized that I had been experiencing them and losing myself in different core feelings every day. No wonder I felt exhausted. I had all these messages and rules that silently directed my whole life. I always felt I wasn't worthy; I felt hopeless and stupid."

When asked when those core feelings began, she realized they started when, as a child, she was sexually abused by a friend of the family. That made sense to Annie, but surprised her because she could very clearly remember deciding "something like that could affect everyone else, but not me. I willed it away."

This woman who appeared to have it all together was never happy with herself. She may have been determined that the abuse would not affect her, but those core feelings remained as its residue. That feeling influenced her significantly as she developed into an adult. She related, "Until I realized that these feelings were con-nected to the past, I didn't think there was anything I could do to change how I felt about myself. When I discovered that my life did actually make sense, I immediately felt I wasn't stupid. I began to see that I had choices, and just knowing that took me out of feeling trapped and hopeless—two core feelings that I now know I can stop."

That knowledge began a change in how Annie thought about herself. She realized she had the opportunity not only to stop these feelings from leading her to food but also to circumvent those serious roadblocks to her feeling secure and satisfied with herself. She was able to start chipping away at her core feelings. Although she would need to continue working to further decrease their power, she had made an essential powerful move for herself.

Like Annie, you can gain an immediate ability to change your feelings by taking the following steps:

1. Recognize core feelings when they occur.
2. Use grounding techniques to focus and stop dissociation.
3. Identify the core messages you give yourself.
4. Ask yourself when you first remember those core feelings and messages occurring.
5. Do not delve deeply into the traumatic experience or loss when you are having a core feeling, but stay with it long enough to acknowledge that your core feelings made sense at the time.
6. Look at the core feelings and recognize that, just by taking these few steps, you have already started to take away their power.

More Stories of Success

One of the most important aspects of letting go of the past is recognizing that you are not alone in your struggle. Reading others' stories provides encouragement so that, whatever your background or history, you can use the same tools others have successfully used to move forward with your life.

In the following stories, highlight parts that remind you of yourself. How you use food may differ, but you may have feelings or circumstances in common.

Bill

Bill, a young accountant, long ago gave up on losing weight and keeping it off for any length of time. He claimed he needed to lose weight now only because of a medical condition, the only way he could justify trying one more time to conquer what he considered his personal failure. Like many others, Bill had underlying issues that contributed to his battle with the pounds. He had suffered from an enormous amount of loss. Recognizing the impact of those losses and his feel-ings of abandonment is an important passage for men like Bill, who were trained as boys not to acknowledge any feeling except power. When Bill began to recognize the relationship of these issues to his eating behaviors, he became intrigued by the process of getting to know himself. Hesitant at first to believe, he simply absorbed himself in progressing through the steps and working the exercises to end his reliance on food.

With the reassurance he felt by reading others' stories, Bill was able to let go of a considerable amount of pain and loss in his life. He could also trace the origin of his use of food back almost to the time the pain began. He said, holding back tears, "I remember the first time my mother told me I was a mistake. I remember like I was stand-ing in front of her today. She looked at me with those cold, steely eyes. Her words just reinforced what she had demonstrated to me since the day I was born.

"I ran outside to get away. I spent a lot of time as a child wan-dering the small town where we lived. A lady down the street saw me and invited me in to have fresh cookies. My gosh, I was only five. I remember stuffing myself and stuffing some cookies in my pockets to eat later. I ate them on my way home. There was no way I was going to share them with my mother. I didn't realize how much that affected me until today. That was a pretty lousy thing for a mother to do. I felt so alone, so wrong."

With help, Bill realized those were his exact feelings before he medicated with binges as an adult. After having that recognition, he used grounding techniques the next time the feeling flashback occurred. He stopped what previously would have been a chain reac-tion into the Cycle of Pain by using reality checks, self talk, and self-affirmations, all tools you'll learn in the next chapter. Since he no longer needed food to get out of those feelings, his overeating stopped, and the pounds began to come off.

Mickey

Mickey could not pinpoint when he began to have a problem with his weight. It seemed as if one day he had awakened with an extra thirty pounds. He attributed it to not being as athletic as he was when he was younger. He claimed he did not eat between meals, yet snack food wrappers were often scattered on the back seat of his car. When stress escalated, Mickey's wife noticed that her husband ate faster and more frequently. He had a caretaking personality and accepted responsibility for many things beyond his control. As a result, he often felt inadequate. He felt that he was a failure, but he did not express those feelings to anyone. He ate them away.

Mickey's life had changed years ago. His father committed suicide, and Mickey blamed himself for not stopping it. He assumed responsibility for someone he loved abandoning him. He began to bury these overwhelming feelings of guilt with food. Guilt kept him from taking time to engage in sports. The core feeling of being a failure for not saving his father's life kept him from many challenges. Food kept buried that part of him that felt out of control. However, whenever he was triggered by similar feelings in his life, his food intake increased. Nothing changed except his weight. He continued to carry feelings that hurt and kept him from progressing. When Mickey addressed these with the steps you're learning now, he not only stopped using food as an emotional blindfold, but he also experienced new freedom in other areas of his life. He was no longer frozen in fear. As he worked to shed his emotional weight, his physical weight quickly stabilized. When he successfully took apart and stopped his progression into the Cycle of Pain, Mickey began walking, eating more healthfully, and actually losing pounds he didn't gain back.

Celia

As triggers to her Cycle of Pain, Celia identified feelings of being used, being alone in the world, and not being good enough. She was a professional woman who often overextended herself, took on other people's responsibilities, and felt frustrated and inept because she did not have time to complete all her assignments. She did not think she lived up to her employer's expectations and believed her husband when he told her she was not a good enough mother, wife, or housekeeper.

Celia felt all alone, even in her marriage. The minute she walked in the door at home, she reverted to her coping mechanism of going numb, of going through the motions. She waited until her husband was asleep, then slipped into the bathroom to take several laxatives to purge her body. Her whole being was focused on getting rid of the overwhelming fat she felt every moment of the day. She knew that checking the scale several times tomorrow would tell her if she were successful and how to feel, and would bring some temporary relief. Now she did not feel alone. Bulimia had become a comfortable friend to ease her pain. It was something she felt in control of and could do "right." Celia, too, was far removed from acknowledging the origins of her problems, which by now had progressed into an eating disorder. Every time she attempted to make progress, old messages and feelings blocked her.

Celia long ago began to rely on others to tell her how to feel. Her self-esteem was built upon pleasing people who could not accept her for the kind, caring woman she was. Until she broke free of that fragile dependency, her relationships at home and work were driven by guilt, by a sense of being rejected, and by never being good enough. Celia said, "I think I continued bingeing, using laxatives, and then not eating for days because the eating disorder was the only thing that was really mine; I could rely on it and it made me feel special. No one could really control me. It was only when it got so out of control that I became so frightened."

She acknowledged that, while the purging often immediately eased her anxiety, soon after, she would feel the familiar overwhelming shame, and then guilt. Guilt would turn into depression. Her Cycle of Pain continued until Celia worked herself into another purge. What started as a once-a-week method to ease the anxiety was now up to three times a day and sometimes more.

Celia wanted to believe her eating disorder did not affect her, but a girlfriend's loving words pointed out to her that its consequences included major work problems, including trouble focusing, forgetfulness, confusion, starting projects she never finished, and a general lack of energy.

Celia confided, "When I first talked about giving it up, I was terrified. I didn't know anything else existed. I thought if I gave it up, there would be nothing there but a black hole.

"It was only after I learned about why I had been using food and purging that I became much stronger emotionally. It wasn't so scary because then I was able to get out of being flooded with my feelings long enough to face my problems head-on. I began using the steps to build up my self-confidence and found I gradually was not dependent upon others to tell me how I should feel or who I am."

It Takes Tools, Not Willpower

As you've seen, willpower alone is not enough for you to maintain a healthy, satisfying weight range. In the next chapter, you'll learn hands-on techniques to fight back, not only at the intrusion of trauma bonds but at anything else that is interfering with your sense of security and with how you feel about yourself. In exploring trauma bonds, you've opened the door to a new understanding of yourself that is not limited by the judgments and hurrahs of past weight loss programs. You've accomplished some of the most difficult work and, in doing so, have learned new tools that can help you not only with the past but in moving through any other struggles you may encounter in life.

AFFIRMATION

My experiences are my teachers. In acknowledging my past,
I can mold harmony and security into my future.

4

BURNING
SELF-TALK GARBAGE

*Our life is what
our thoughts make of it.*
—Marcus Aurelius

Somewhere in the background of every person with chronic weight struggles lies a trash heap of rigorous, righteous core messages: shoulds, shouldn'ts, and other such junk. These messages frequently trigger destructive eating behaviors. You already have begun to notice messages that precipitate changes in your mood. Ultimately, these messages become internalized and deprive you of a chance to feel good about yourself. Whatever the reason for the development of these messages, you pay the price until the messages are stopped. In this chapter, you'll start to change the internalized core message, and burn your self-talk garbage.

Step 3: Burn your negative self-talk garbage.
When you stop your negative self-talk, you'll stop turning the power of your emotions over to others. In this chapter, you'll learn about talkback, reality checks, and affirmations—all tools to use to put the power of your emotions back where it belongs: with you.

Shovel Out What You Put In
Simply by recognizing how many messages trigger intense reactions, you gain control over them. Initially, it can be somewhat over-

whelming. Just remember, you have lived with some of these messages for a lifetime, and it will take concerted effort to discard them.

Messages become automatic. Sometimes it seems as if no matter what anyone says, it hurts. If someone doesn't read your mind to know something you want to hear, that hurts. You fill in the blanks to destroy any good feelings about yourself. This is a learned response and can be changed.

In the following exercise, think about how often you give yourself negative messages, and then think about how much energy you will have when you stop the destructive self talk. Circle the self-destructive messages that trigger your use of food.

Identifying Self-Destructive Messages

1. I can't do anything right.
2. If I lost weight, there wouldn't be any problems in my . . .
3. I should . . .
4. I need to . . .
5. If I just tried harder, I could (lose weight, get it right) . . .
6. If I lost weight, my whole life would change.
7. I am not worthy of a good relationship.
8. I have to do (produce) more.
9. I'm not good enough.
10. I don't have a right to complain.
11. I need someone to take care of me.
12. If I don't control everything, I will be hurt.
13. It is more important to prevent others from being hurt than to protect myself.
14. All people see when they look at me is fat.
15. There is something wrong with me.
16. I don't want to be in a confrontation.

List other messages you use to sabotage yourself.

1. _____

2. _____

3. _____

Add to the list as you proceed through your journey. Then attack each negative message with the tools you're learning. You've already learned some tools to use, such as grounding techniques. Continue to use those, along with these new ones: talking back, reality checks, and affirmations. We'll look at each one in detail. Beginning with Step 1, you'll examine how these negative messages work against you today; then with Step 2, you'll learn how to face down this self-destruction head-on with strong talkback; and finally in Step 3, you'll learn to safeguard yourself against emotional food use by using reality checks as powerful responses to meet your needs.

1. Identifying Bad Core Messages

Does your garbage pile of negative messages make you feel good or bad?

Close your eyes for a moment and picture a little child. Think of your negative self-talk messages. Describe, by talking aloud or writing, how a child would feel as he or she hears your negative messages. How do you think you may have felt when you first heard them? Next, consider your feelings as an adult when you have been made vulnerable by loss or circumstances. Are those the same feelings you experience today before eating or not eating?

Use writing or art to express your feelings. Then make a copy of the following chart. List the connections you made, and add to the chart as you progress through the book.

The next part in identifying your bad core messages is a type of self-parenting: focus on what you felt when you heard one of your own core messages, then note how you would empathetically respond to a child or vulnerable adult in that same circumstance. For example, if you come upon a child who feels worthless because he is consistently told he can't do anything right, how would you provide

Identifying Messages That Trigger Eating		
When I hear those messages, I feel...	How did the child feel? Or, how did the vulnerable adult feel?	What feelings/ messages trigger destructive eating?

solace to that child? Or, if you could comfort someone whose husband told her he was leaving her because of her weight, what would you do to ease her pain? Think of what you would say and what you would do. Now give yourself that same gentle nurturing.

Finally, reflect on your progress so far. First, you stopped yourself from overreacting and analyzed what was happening with the thinking part of your brain. Second, you closed your eyes and visualized your situation, which not only tapped into the creative part of your brain but also pulled in your heart. Third, you used writing and art, which continued the process of integrating your head and heart to absorb what you have learned. Fourth, you developed a concrete reference tool to keep as a reminder—a cheat sheet of sorts. Finally, you sat quietly with what you learned and provided yourself with emotional support that is not dependent upon another person. This technique balances your emotions and thinking.

At this point, you have begun to change your beliefs about yourself. Instead of thinking it is hopeless to change those old negative thoughts and patterns, you understand now how they are connected. Therefore, you know they can be taken apart.

For example, while the third column of the Identifying Messages chart may seem repetitive, it provides needed reinforcement. It is your light bulb. It not only shows that you have made a clear connection and, therefore, have begun the process of change, but also that your responses in the past made sense at the time, based on what happened. Remember, you're making positive changes for yourself because you've jumped into the exercises willing to actively explore your unique history, carefully considering how it has affected you and challenging yourself to make changes, step by step, as you gather more information and tools. Each component of these exercises is built to reinforce a long-lasting change, not just to create a momentary reflection.

Lastly, in completing the exercise process, you identified messages that have significantly impacted your life, not only by triggering unhealthful eating but by limiting your potential. Give these messages special attention as you complete the remainder of the exercises in the book.

Pat yourself on the back. You have increased your understanding and gained a sense of control in how you feel about yourself. Just identifying your own personal garbage messages can stop you from using food. Or, it may slow down what was once an immediate trigger to eating until you learn more ways to intervene. Either way, it is another piece of that puzzle that will help you end your reliance on food. In the next section, you'll learn more proactive steps to stop the negative influences of those old messages.

2. Talking Back at Your Core Messages

Now that you've progressed through the first step to burn the garbage by identifying self-destructive messages, you're ready to dig deeper. The second step is to stop the messages from interfering with your life. You'll learn how to tune into and eliminate that chatterbox in your head.

You are giving yourself permission to talk back—to be heard. What you say is important! Children who develop food and weight issues often are taught their side of the story is not important. They may feel stupid or not entitled to talk as an adult. Or, when they talk, they may find themselves always on the defensive. Adults may not talk for the same reason, or they may not speak out for fear someone will think they are looking for pity, or they may feel they do not have the right to speak up to anyone in authority. Take action if you hear a message in your head that sabotages you. Say aloud, *Stop! That's a bunch of baloney!*

Talking back is simply standing up for yourself. It is a way you can stop cold a thought process that often is blaming and self-persecutory. It allows you time to think about a situation and not feel pressured. It helps you eliminate hammering thoughts that make you feel lousy with no justification. It helps break the drive for food when you hurt and don't know what else to do.

You want to blast an irrational thought out of your mind with forceful, directive words. Don't try to be too nice! You need to get your own attention because you have become used to piling on negative thoughts. Think of what you would say to a friend, and treat yourself just as well. For example, if you say, "I'm bad because I ate that cake," your talkback statement might be: "That's ridiculous! Eating a piece of cake doesn't make me bad inside. It is just food." Or, if you start to feel that you can never do anything good enough after you receive a B instead of an A on a report card, tell yourself: "That's nuts! I worked hard for that B, and it is a good grade. I've got to stop beating myself up. That grade is good enough." Note that you're not saying "I'm nuts" or "I'm stupid" for thinking that way. If you did, you would be reinforcing core feelings or negative self talk and certainly wouldn't feel any better. Always be on the lookout for what you are saying to yourself, because those words are totally in your control and you are the only one who has the power to change how you think about yourself.

While you're talking back to yourself, move! Physical movement such as snapping your fingers, tapping furniture, or stomping your feet help remove you from the intense feeling and pull you into taking action to replace it. With practice, it becomes easier to talk back to your negative messages, as you would talk back to anyone who had offended someone you love.

3. Serving Yourself a Reality Check (Instead of Food)

Freedom comes when you begin to experience increased feelings of serenity without using food. Using reality checks is a huge step toward that serenity.

We all persecute ourselves from time to time with junk messages; for purposes of example, let's look at the messages you might get if you had grown up in a troubled family. In a troubled family, you may have been taught not to believe reality. The family system would fall apart if you did. You learned not to cry when you were hurt, or to cry excessively because it was the only means to get attention for your hurt. You may have learned that it was okay to be hurt by an authority figure or by someone you love or that it was not safe to visibly or verbally rebel too much. Perhaps you learned to rebel quietly, with control of food. Eating or not eating. Hiding, or even stealing food.

Pretty soon you learned to believe what was said: that you are stupid, ugly, fat, or lazy. Simply put, you learned to adapt to your environment to survive. If that meant absorbing negative messages, that is what you did (and still do). Those messages definitely affected your emotional development. They continue to haunt and confuse you as an adult. They hold power today, whether they are from someone else or are self-inflicted. The messages shatter a sense of control and can propel you toward the use of food to feel better. Is it any wonder a diet alone could not combat that?

Reality checks are crucial, no matter what your background, when someone says something that makes you feel hurt or threatened or when you hear the voice of persecution within your own head. First, say *No!* every time you hear a persecutory thought instead of automatically absorbing its contents. This negation will allow your thoughts to slow as you ask yourself specific questions, which you'll read about in the next section. Instead of automatically assuming the worst about yourself, learn to question the motives and reality of those who put you down—including yourself!

During the next few weeks, make a note every time you use the following techniques. Include a description of the situation, the specific techniques you used, how you felt after, and how your action helped you change how you think about yourself. Don't beat yourself up if you have missed opportunities or have been fearful to use the techniques you've learned earlier in this chapter. It's all part of the learning process. As with any exercise in *Body Sense*, just analyze how you could handle the same situation next time. You may want to practice the response you would have liked to make in front of a mirror, or write it down. Always address the situation in some way, even if the opportunity for immediate action is gone. You'll still benefit from the practice and will be more confident the next time.

Reality Check Techniques

- Assume that a negative message is not true until you have specific proof.
- Ask specific questions. When? Where? What behavior? Do not ask Why questions. These tend to become more philosophical, and it becomes easier for you to be distracted from the present.
- Consider the person. Does someone have a motive for making you feel a certain way? Is there a purpose behind the negative message? What would you reply if someone else that you weren't emotionally involved with said that same thing to you? How would you recommend a friend respond, if someone said that to her? Do you treat yourself as well as you treat a friend? Are you reacting to this person in a certain way because something about the person reminds you of someone else?
- Don't accept generalizations. It is impossible to address general messages that are undefined and insurmountable. Always work to get to the bottom of the messages so you can determine what really is the issue. If someone says you are out of control, ask for specifics. "When specifically did you see that behavior?"

- Become a broken record. Most domineering people will beat a subject to death until you give in because of your fatigue, frustration, or sometimes a sense of hopelessness. Eventually, they will wear down defenses as they target another vulnerable area. Repeat your facts. If the person does not respond to the facts, conclude the conversation, or you will be pulled into their reality. There is nothing to be gained by such conversation. You do not have to prove anything.

- Ask yourself if you are overreacting to what was said. Did what was said spark a feelings flashback and start the Cycle of Pain?

- Take a moment to consider whether or not you are overreacting because of a trauma bond or because the person speaking to you is being unkind. Your feelings are occurring for a reason. If you determine you are reacting to a trauma bond, you know it is important to go back and analyze where it is anchored. Then use the other exercises in this chapter to combat its recurrence. If the person is being rude or controlling, it is reasonable that you will react. However, you can control that reaction by using the tools you will learn, in this chapter, and especially with the assertiveness techniques you'll learn in chapter 8, "Make Anger Work for You."

- If, after slowing your reaction, you agree with that person's reality, you can take steps to change—if you want.

- Ask yourself if you are reacting with fear. Ask, "What is the worst thing that can happen if what I am afraid of occurs? What is the best thing that can happen?" Then answer as truthfully as possible. For example: What is the worst thing that can happen if I binge after I enter the recovery journey? I would use it to reinforce a sense of failure and as an excuse not to go on. What is the best thing that can happen? I would connect the feelings I had before the binge to the behavior and work to eliminate that trigger's power. I would accept this as a learning experience and acknowledge that I am a human being who does not have to be perfect.

4. Replacing Your Negative Messages

Using what you have learned about talkback and reality checks, formulate replacement messages for each negative message. Your new messages should be believable to you right now. Later, you may expand upon them. Every day, replace negative messages as they invade your thinking. It is important you replace *every* garbage message with a new message: you are chipping away at an old belief system—one that hasn't worked.

If a message causes you intense pain, recognize its impact and begin to tune into how much that message seeps into your thinking process. Does it affect your feelings and actions? It may surprise you. The message and corresponding feeling may be a powerful trigger in your using food as a destructive force. That cycle also can contribute to ongoing unhappiness and lack of satisfaction.

If you begin to absorb the garbage messages, stop. Make the decision to protect yourself when you feel uncomfortable or uneasy. This decision is an important step in your recovery. Your feelings are legitimate. You also have a choice to complete the exercise later.

Exercise: Search and Destroy Your Junk Messages

The following exercise will help you systematically discard messages that you use against yourself today. Write the message down exactly as you hear it in your head. Your power comes in disassembling your exact message. Then replace it with a message you can believe today. Don't make it pie-in-the-sky. Make the message straightforward and listen to it. As the old messages die away, you will find the pounds will come off easier. Here's an example:

Junk Message: You cannot make a decision on your own. It will always be wrong.

Replacement Message: I am making the decisions I need to make right now. No one can always be right. I can choose to allow myself to make a mistake and move on.

Here are some more junk messages that may be similar to your own. For each, write down an empowering replacement message, and then, after you're warmed up, write down your own junk messages, either now or as they occur to you later.

Junk Message: No matter what you do, it is not good enough.

Replacement Message:

Junk Message: You are overweight. Therefore no one will like you.

Replacement Message:

Junk Message: There is something wrong with you.

Replacement Message:

Junk Message: I'm doing this only for your own good.

Replacement Message:

Junk Message: No one will ever love you the way I do.

Replacement Message:

Junk Message:

Replacement Message:

Junk Message:

Replacement Message:

Junk Message:

Replacement Message:

Well done! Consider how much emotional energy you're going to have as you continue to discard those old junk messages!

5. Affirming Yourself to Wholeness

Affirmations replace negative messages with positive ones of hope. Start with simple, positive statements. As in your new messages to yourself, don't make the affirmations grandiose. For instance, what person unhappy with weight could believe this statement: "I have a beautiful body"? Millions of defense mechanisms would begin working! However, that same person may believe this affirmation: "My body is only a part of who I am." Make the affirmation fit your need now: nothing fancy, nothing far-fetched, just a thought that will become a reality as you incorporate it daily into your life. The wonderful thing is that, for every negative message, there is an affirmation. Here are two examples:

Negative Message: What I say is not important. I'm not important.
Affirmation: I have a right to be heard.

Negative Message: I am different from my family. I must be crazy. Something must be wrong with me.
Affirmation: I am a unique person. I can make my own decisions. I am different and sane. It feels good to be different from my family.

Effectively using affirmations takes practice. The payoff is worth the work, however, because eventually you will internalize them. No, they don't work all the time or every time you feel unhappy about yourself. They don't work all the time for anyone. However, affirmations and talkback are powerful tools that will work effectively most of the time for you.

6. Making Affirmations and Talkback Work

Copy your affirmations onto index cards and take them with you wherever you go. Nourish yourself by looking at them several times during the day—more if a situation is particularly stressful. Make affirmation breaks as regular as coffee breaks.

You may find it helpful to copy the negative message on one half of the card and the talkback message on the other half. Then flip the card over and represent your affirmation in words or pictures on the other side. This approach helps you connect all three parts of the process.

Use every opportunity to reinforce what you are learning. It takes repeated actions to replace an old belief system with one sparkling with confidence and positive beliefs about yourself. Think for a moment, how else can you use affirmations? For example, you may want to begin by adding your own affirmation to the one that is included at the end of each chapter. Or, you may decide to make writing an affirmation a daily gift to yourself. Use the following examples as a jumping-off point to form your own affirmations that strike back at your junk talk.

Negative Message: If I lost weight, my husband would not divorce me.
Talkback: No. I'm not taking all the blame. My husband has significant problems. He blames everything on me so he can justify an affair.
Affirmation: I am more than just my weight. I am a whole person.

Negative Message: My body is repulsive.
Talkback: Stop. I am learning why I feel this way, and I can change.
Affirmation: My body is only part of who I am. Or (a more direct attack): I can accept my _____ today (pick one part of your body that you can accept today).

Negative Message:

Talkback:

Affirmation:

On a separate sheet of paper, write down as many negative messages, talkbacks, and affirmations as you can think of. Each time you hear a new message, write it down and attack it! With practice, you'll soon find that talkbacks, reality checks, and affirmations have become your natural response to every negative message.

7. Accepting Positives from the Past

Is our pile of core messages from our past all bad? Of course not! In most cases, childhood wasn't full of negative messages. However, because the negative ones can be overwhelming, the positive messages are often misplaced. Another problem is that positive and negative messages often come from the same person and so both kinds are believed. Adults other than parents may also provided positives. Teachers, a friend's mother, or an aunt may have encouraged you. Some children get encouragement from books. Take a moment to recall positive messages you carry with you. Are you using them frequently to provide self-encouragement? Make a note of these below, as reminders for you on days when you need to provide yourself with a few kind words.

Positive Messages I Carry with Me Today:

1. _____
2. _____
3. _____

Persistence Pays Off

Burning your self-talk garbage will take time. But you have already reduced your vulnerability by walking through this process, and you will know how to tackle problems in the future without the use of food as a support.

Each time you identify a garbage message and the accompanying feeling in the coming week, note the action you take on the following chart. Think for a moment of what you might have done in the past and how you have made positive changes that ultimately will

Action to Unload the Garbage

Date	Garbage Message	Feeling	Action Taken (Talkback, Reality Checks, Grounding Techniques, Movement, Affirmation)	Replacement Feeling

replace using food. Congratulate yourself. Although some of these messages have been absorbed over a lifetime, you have already begun to make them crumble.

When you have unloaded the garbage, a tremendous weight will be off your shoulders. As you have learned, emotional weight translates into pounds. In the next chapter, you're going to take a compassionate look at difficult times in your life when you may have neglected your needs, simply because you may have felt you would fall apart if you owned the intensity of your feelings, or you felt that others' feelings were more important.

Now that you are allowing yourself time and have learned the importance of honoring your own feelings, you'll be able to address your needs immediately. Therefore, you'll have no reason to push away your feelings with food. Since you have already begun to make crucial links between your use of food and the pain anchored to the past, you'll also recognize the need to honor those feelings and attack any garbage messages that remain anchored.

Work hard and have patience with yourself. Remember, learning is absorbed one small step at a time. Recognize the importance of each step and applaud yourself. Movement is important. While it may have taken years for these junk messages to have become a part of your belief system, you now have the tools to make them go away.

AFFIrmATIon
I can make the most powerful changes
in the world within myself.

5

Rx FOR EMOTIONAL EATING: IDENTIFY YOUR FEELINGS

This above all: to thine own self be true, and
it must follow, as the night the day, thou canst
not then be false to any man.

—William Shakespeare

Cookies really can make you feel better, at least for awhile.

Food alters your mood. Eating or not eating may temporarily take away the pain. For brief periods, you may feel in control, satisfied, or relieved from constant pressures. You may even feel a surge of self-esteem, power, or comfort.

As you have learned, abuse of food is often born to numb out when your feelings put you into overload. When you acknowledge your feelings as they are experienced, you'll react appropriately in a timely manner rather than becoming overwhelmed with those feelings later and reacting ineffectively because you no longer have a direct connection with the cause.

Step 4: Identify your feelings and analyze their purpose; then take appropriate actions to care for yourself.
This step is the foundation for understanding why you use food to change feelings, and it will provide you with a strong base to communicate more assertively. By identifying the patterns that reinforce eating behaviors, you can then take action to intervene. It would be like taking acetaminophen to reduce a fever: when you have the knowledge, it becomes your choice whether to use it. One

prescription you already began in chapter 3 is to identify the feelings associated with your eating. This awareness will help you break the Cycle of Pain and begin a new Cycle of Health. Each time you intervene to change an old behavior, you gain more strength and momentum.

This identifying process can be difficult initially, because you probably have successfully numbed your feelings for some time, perhaps because you do not like conflict or because you are afraid of your feelings or of others' reactions to them. Maybe you're worried that your feelings may hurt others. Perhaps you do not think your feelings are valid or important. If you have blocked your feelings, it may be difficult to acknowledge them, unless you consider it a good feeling. Remember, there are no good or bad feelings. Each feeling has a purpose: your job is to listen to what the feeling is telling you. That doesn't mean automatically acting upon your feeling. As you have learned, sometimes feelings from the past flood us and cause distortions. Listen to your feeling, think about the message you are getting from it, and consider what action it is prompting you to take. Then consider your options.

You may want to make a copy of the Feelings Short List that follows and stick it in your pocket, initially, as you begin to tune in and connect your feelings with your food use. If you are in a situation and feel unaware, numb, or extremely intense, make sure you push yourself to describe at least three other feelings. You'll find that will pull you out of the numbness or feelings flashback and allow you to take care of yourself. If you don't stop for this moment of self-reflection, you may acknowledge only the feeling you are most comfortable with and neglect to take appropriate action on the others. Notice that "bored" is not on this list, although it is on the longer list that follows. That's because you may say you are eating because you are bored, thereby neglecting to express any deeper or apparently unacceptable feelings and pushing those feelings down, not accepting the message they are sending.

For the next few days, carry this list. Refer to it frequently, especially during any stressful situation. Then ask yourself, what do I need to do with this feeling? Is it prompting me to some action? If you're headed toward the kitchen, you are going to alleviate the feeling only temporarily. Use what you've learned about trauma bonds and burning your garbage to help you further decide what your next step will be, once you have connected to your true feelings.

Feelings Short List

Anger	Guilt	Rage
Fear	Happiness	Shame

You will also want to make several copies of the following longer feelings list, which is more descriptive. Put one on your refrigerator, or use it in your journal as a starting point as you take your emotional temperature each day.

Feelings List

Abandoned	Contentment	Exasperated
Accepted	Decrease in function	Fear
Afraid	Defective	Flooded with feelings
Alarmed	Defiant	Foolish
Alone	Delighted	Free
Anger	Depressed	Frightened
Annoyed	Deprived	Frozen
Anticipation	Desire	Fulfilled
Anxious	Desolate	Glad
Apprehensive	Despondent	Guilt
Ashamed	Dirty	Happy
Belonging	Disappointment	Hate
Betrayed	Eager	Helpless
Chagrined	Embarrassed	Hopeless
Confident	Empty	Hostile

Humiliated	Need to be punished	Self-pity
Hungry	Nervous	Shy
Hurt	Not good enough	Soiled
Inadequate	Overwhelmed	Sorrowful
Incapable	Pain	Stupid
Incomplete	Peaceful	Suspicious
Indebted to someone	Pleasure	Terror
Insufficient	Punishing	Threatened
Irritated	Rage	Timid
Joyous	Relief	Uneasy
Lacking	Rejected	Unhappy
Longing	Remorse	Unloved
Lost	Resentment	Unwanted
Loved	Responsible	Wanting
Low spirits	Sad	Weak
Melancholic	Satisfied	Withdrawn
Needy	Serene	Worthless

As you increase your ability to listen to your feelings, you may want to continue to carry a copy of the longer feelings list. Don't be overwhelmed by the number of feelings on the list. Each is a description of different shades of feelings that were on the short list. The longer feelings list helps you to further define these shades.

Check your feelings at least four times each day. Take it slowly. You may not have been tuned into the range of your feelings before. For instance, you may have thought you were eating because you were bored, but you really were eating because you also were hurt or angry. Because you medicated those feelings with food, you cheated yourself out of an opportunity to take action to eliminate them. But now, as you identify feelings, you will be able to make the connection between your feelings and your cravings for certain foods, your impulse to binge, or your impulse to abstain from eating. Making this connection is an important step to true long-term healing.

Since you're recognizing the variety of feelings you experience daily, the next step is to connect them closely to your use of food. Make a copy of the Recognizing My Feelings chart that follows, and write down at least four feelings each day for a week or two. Then note the trigger to those feelings, and decide whether you used food in reaction. At the bottom of the chart, note any patterns you see emerging.

Recognizing My Feelings				
	Time	Feeling	Trigger	Did I think of food?
Monday				
Tuesday				
Wednesday				
Thursday				
Friday				
Saturday				
Sunday				

Patterns I want to investigate:

Now that you have started to own your feelings, use the next chart to analyze which ones are more likely to trigger you into unhealthful eating. Make an extra copy and use it for the next two weeks, adding to it each time you think about food, have a craving, eat, or engage in self-destructive use of food. It might be helpful to use checkmarks as you go or to carry it one step further and put the

Feelings Connection Chart

These feelings make me crave food, want to binge, purge, not eat, or obsessively exercise.

	Never	Rarely	Sometimes	Frequently	Always
Abandoned					
Anger					
Anxiety					
Betrayal					
Boredom					
Consolation					
Control					
Depression					
Deprivation					
Distraction					
Embarrassment/ Humiliation					
Empty					
Fear/Terror					
Hunger					
Ignored					
Incapable					
Loneliness					
Low self-esteem					
Numb					
Overwhelmed					
Power					
Punishment					
Rebellion					
Reward					
Stress					
Unimportant					
Unloved					

initial of what you actually do, for example, c for craving, o for overeating, and so on.

From Identifying Feelings to Changing Feelings

Once you identify why you are using food, you can begin to use the tools you've learned. For example, if you discover you are eating because you are feeling deprived, use reality checks grounding techniques, and then, if needed, explore the possibility that you may be overreacting because of a trauma bond. When you sort that out, you can then also use tools like talkback and affirmations to attack destructive messages.

The next time you have a feeling that precipitates eating, *stop*! Think about what you *really* need. For example, if you feel incapable, you need some method totally under your control to make you feel capable. In chapter 4, you learned about reality checks, talkback, and affirmations; all will combat that feeling. If you are feeling fear, do something to make you safe. That means removing yourself from a dangerous environment, or stepping back to assess where your feelings of emotional reaction came from. You've already learned that fear can be connected to a trauma bond, and in chapters 3 and 4 you've learned ways to begin to break that bond. In chapter 6, you'll learn more about how these feelings prompt messages and how you can take control just by changing what you say to yourself. You're learning one step at a time to make lasting changes. You're also gaining increasing control as you identify what emotional triggers, or feelings, push you to or away from food. Instead of using food to alter feelings, you're beginning to embrace feelings as messengers that give you clues to determine your next steps in staying healthy and happy.

Prescriptions to Put You in Control

As we've seen, in the Cycle of Pain, there is an endless pattern of feelings triggering destructive eating. Small interventions in this cycle ultimately build to put the brakes on this damaging behavior.

Two additional intervention techniques are the Food and Feelings Monitor Form and the Food Diary described below. Both will heighten your awareness of your use of food to moderate feelings. They'll also help you identify your triggers to the destructive use of food. When these triggers are identified, other interventions can be used to reduce their power.

These charts are only tools. They are not meant to shame you into stopping your behaviors. You are the only one who has to see them. You know you are in charge, and anything you do is a choice. If you decide not to do an exercise, think about why. That may be as important to your transformation as completing a chart. However, the more you complete, the stronger you are making the statement that you are important and that you will take the time to get to know yourself.

Make enough copies of the daily Food Diary for two to four weeks. If you do not eat, fill one out anyway for that meal time. Add any in-between snacks, too.

Exercise: Food Diary

Feelings and attitude upon awakening _____

Breakfast: Time _____Place _____With whom _____

Feelings before eating _____Feelings during meal _____

Feelings after eating _____

Lunch: Time _____Place _____With whom _____

Feelings before eating _____Feelings during meal _____

Feelings after eating _____

Dinner: Time_____Place _____With whom _____

Feelings before eating _____Feelings during meal _____

Feelings after eating _____

Snack: Time _____Place _____With whom _____

Feelings before eating _____Feelings during meal _____

Feelings after eating _____

Feelings and attitude at end of day _____

As time passes, look for important patterns. For instance, if you discover that you are stopping to eat on your way home, you may be trying to soothe anxiety about facing problems at home. What feelings besides hunger led you to eat? What feelings followed during and after eating? Are there more efficient ways you can attain those same feelings? Did you notice how time and place are also connected to your eating? Does eating alone or with a particular person increase or decrease your food intake? If so, you'll want to continue to analyze and take actions on issues surrounding that environment or your relationships.

Owning Your Feelings for Self-Survival

Congratulations! By connecting your feelings with your eating habits, you've begun to differentiate between physical and emotional hunger, a crucial aspect of gaining control of your weight issues. If you have been using food inappropriately to control feelings, you probably eat whether you are hungry or not. Or, if you have chosen to restrict food, you probably have trained yourself to believe you are never hungry.

For the next two to three weeks, use the chart on page 63 to make more important links between your feelings and your eating patterns. For example, by completing column 1, you may discover that you consistently eat at a particular time. Knowing that, you can tune into what typically goes on during your day at that time. Or, by completing column 2, you may find that eating a particular type of food triggers a binge. In chapter 9, you'll learn more about the chemical impacts of certain foods. Of course, it is important to tune into your physical hunger level by completing column 3. Once you identify the specific feeling you are trying to eliminate in column 4, you can determine whether you are accurately reacting to something in the present or whether you are overreacting to a core feeling that originated long ago. In that case, it would be more efficient for you to stop and work to break a trauma bond, use reality checks, or apply other methods to take care of that feeling. From your response in column 5, you'll know you need to work on alternative ways to get that same positive feeling. Recognizing a precipitating event in column 6 can help you gain more control in actively attacking issues that keep you connected to the Cycle of Pain. You can take it apart to analyze what particular aspect caused an emotional reaction. You may want to write in your journal about it, or talk to a friend. Look for overreactions to core feelings, misperceptions, and self-blame. Then use reality checks and the techniques you've learned to attack junk messages.

Make copies and use this chart for two to three weeks. Each week, analyze its contents to determine what needs more focus.

Pain Triggers

You may have found that you reach for food after contact with a particular person who activates deeply buried core feelings or intense feelings based on misperceptions. While you may not immediately search out food, the contact may push you back into the Cycle of Pain, which in the past has led you back to food. Recognizing that pattern will help you identify specific core feelings and relationships that you'll still want to focus on. Often the feeling is related to the person you are talking with, but it also may be a core feeling that is easily activated and can create an environment of misperceptions. For example, if you are still wrestling with a core feeling of feeling stupid, you might overreact if your mother consistently offers unsolicited advice. You may be allowing her to do this by not setting your boundaries, with the result being that you misperceive her intent and message. When you set boundaries with your mother, it will get you closer to examining whatever connection there remains to that core feeling of stupid. Or your feeling may be anchored to a painful experience with someone else that you were unable to explore until you had proven to yourself that you had the strength and ability to set boundaries with someone you love.

Food and Feelings Monitor Chart

Date / Time	Food / Drink	Hunger Level (1–10)*	Feelings before Eating, Restricting, Purging, or Compulsive Exercise	Feelings After	Precipitating Event

* 1: having no hunger / 10: being ravenous.

Your Comments:

Don't be discouraged if you are continuing to uncover core feelings. It is a process similar to peeling the layers of an onion's skin. The more layers you peel away, the more emotional burdens you release. Each level requires you building more strength and confidence in yourself and developing the techniques to be in control of the process.

Examining Perceptions

Perceptions trigger feelings in many ways. If you grew up perceiving you must be perfect, you may have learned not to express your feelings for fear of sounding stupid. If you have gone through a divorce, either as a child or as an adult, you may internalize and blame yourself for someone you love abandoning you. Your message to yourself becomes not to express your feelings because you may lose someone you love. If you have anger or violence in your home, danger may occur when you express feelings. You may have been told that no one would believe you if you expressed your feelings, that your feelings aren't real or important. Or you may have been trained to believe your feelings are selfish or are signs of weakness. If any of these perceptions are true for you, each time you acknowledge a feeling today and for the rest of your life, congratulate yourself for taking control back from the past and standing up for yourself.

The following questionnaire will help determine what triggers still activate your use of food. Add any intense feelings you think may cause you to use your old coping skills. If you find yourself reacting after contact with a specific person, analyze the feeling. Then use reality checks, grounding techniques, and affirmations to take action on any trauma bonds that have been activated. If the triggered feeling is anger, rage, or loss, you'll learn more ways to intervene in chapters 7 and 8.

Triggers Questionnaire

Do I find myself reaching for food after talking to (or seeing) a particular person?

I. After I talk to my mother, I usually feel (circle one)

Empowered   Relief   Comfort   Stable   Alone   Misunderstood
Not good enough   Depressed   Happy   Confident   Inadequate
Angry   Enraged   Empty   Numb   Loss   Dissociated   Hurt
Loved   Unlovable   Unworthy   Fat   Ugly

2. After I talk to my father, I usually feel

Empowered   Relief   Comfort   Stable   Alone   Misunderstood
Not good enough   Depressed   Happy   Confident   Inadequate
Angry   Enraged   Empty   Numb   Loss   Dissociated   Hurt
Loved   Unlovable   Unworthy   Fat   Ugly

3. After I talk to my sibling, I usually feel (complete for each one)

Empowered   Relief   Comfort   Stable   Alone   Misunderstood
Not good enough   Depressed   Happy   Confident   Inadequate
Angry   Enraged   Empty   Numb   Loss   Dissociated   Hurt
Loved   Unlovable   Unworthy   Fat   Ugly

4. After I talk to my significant other, I usually feel

Empowered   Relief   Comfort   Stable   Alone   Misunderstood
Not good enough   Depressed   Happy   Confident   Inadequate
Angry   Enraged   Empty   Numb   Loss   Dissociated   Hurt
Loved   Unlovable   Unworthy   Fat   Ugly

5. After I talk to my friend, I usually feel (complete for each one)

Empowered   Relief   Comfort   Stable   Alone   Misunderstood
Not good enough   Depressed   Happy   Confident   Inadequate
Angry   Enraged   Empty   Numb   Loss   Dissociated   Hurt
Loved   Unlovable   Unworthy   Fat   Ugly

6. After I talk to my boss, I usually feel

Empowered   Relief   Comfort   Stable   Alone   Misunderstood

Not good enough   Depressed   Happy   Confident   Inadequate

Angry   Enraged   Empty   Numb   Loss   Dissociated   Hurt

Loved   Unlovable   Unworthy   Fat   Ugly

Complete the following with anyone else you have consistent contact, such as a coworker or teacher.

7. After I talk to _____, I usually feel

Empowered   Relief   Comfort   Stable   Alone   Misunderstood

Not good enough   Depressed   Happy   Confident   Inadequate

Angry   Enraged   Empty   Numb   Loss   Dissociated   Hurt

Loved   Unlovable   Unworthy   Fat   Ugly

Protecting Yourself from Trigger Feelings

Food is not the only defense for washing away feelings. You, like many people, may use defensive actions—such as laughing or justifying other people's behaviors—when you are hurt, thus running away from the problem. You'll find numerous other actions in the Feelings Defense List that follows. Using these defense mechanisms minimizes your feelings that don't go away with a smile. They may seem easier and less confrontational, but they deprive you of the ability to clearly communicate and get your needs met. These actions tend to interfere with relationships and can be quite destructive, as well as prohibiting you from taking healthier, assertive actions. What begins as protection can become a barrier to getting to know the real you.

During the next week, to make the connections between your eating patterns and your reliance on defenses, use the Food and Feelings Monitor Chart from earlier in the chapter with the Feelings Defense List on the next page. Each time you can connect it with food use, make a note of each defensive action in the margin of the chart.

Feelings Defense List

Agree	Judge
Analyze	Justify
Apologize	Minimize
Attack	Moralize
Be silent	Placate
Complain	Plot revenge
Criticize	Procrastinate
Deny	Project (push your feelings onto
Disagree	someone else)
Evade	Quibble
Explain	Rationalize
Generalize	Run away
Glare	Switch
Go somewhere else in your	Smile
mind: numb, zone out,	Theorize
dissociate	Threaten
Intellectualize	Use sarcasm
Joke	Withdraw

When the week is done, analyze what you have noted. Do you use one defense more than another? Do you notice a connection between an increase in your defensiveness and your use of food? Stay particularly tuned in to what you think, what you say, and how you act when you are being defensive. Since you've also used the Food and Feelings Monitor Chart, you know there are many feelings that may put you on the defensive. If it is a core feeling, you learned in chapter 3 how to stop the chain reaction of a trauma bond by identifying the core feelings and messages and how to begin replacing those negative messages.

Destructive Coping Skills

Now that you've considered how defensive reactions are connected to your use of food, let's consider how other coping skills can be used to escape the intensity of feelings. Circle the unhealthy coping skills you use today. Check the ones you have used in the past.

Coping Skills

As you know, these skills provide only temporary relief, before actually pushing you once again through the Cycle of Pain and, ultimately, back to the inappropriate ways you are using food.

Becoming overly involved
   in taking care of other
   people's problems
Compulsive exercising
Compulsive working, cleaning,
   "doing"
Controlling
Drinking
Engaging in destructive
   relationships
Hiding
Numbing

Overeating
Purging
Sneaking food
Raging
Rationalizing
Rejecting others
Restricting food
Sexually acting out
Sleeping
Using drugs
Withdrawing

In the past five chapters, you've been working hard to recognize feelings when they first occur, to identify their purpose and how they trigger your use of food, and to learn alternative actions to take. Let's summarize the steps you've learned:

1. Acknowledge each feeling is real and has a reason. The reason for its intensity may be much deeper than the event that triggered the pain today.

2. Tell yourself you have a right to feel that way. Give yourself permission to feel as an adult in order to really deal with and rid yourself of the pain.

3. Use grounding techniques. After you acknowledge the pain, orient yourself to the present. Repeat your name, age, and the

fact that you are able to make choices today and take care of yourself today. Snap your fingers or physically move in some way to jolt you out of the past and into today.

4. Share your feeling with a trusted friend, a therapist, or member of a support group. It is important for you to understand you are not alone. Others also have had similar experiences and have changed their lives in positive ways.

5. View the feeling as if you were a reporter. Analyze its possible reasons and causes. This is one way to increase your confidence and decrease your fear of what will happen if you acknowledge hidden feelings.

6. Journal and draw your feelings. This process allows you to use your creative self in conjunction with your intellect to further access positive solutions and clarify your needs. Each action aids in healing and takes you further from using food.

7. Prepare affirmation cards that address the intense feeling. Some affirmations include the following:
   - A child deserves to be loved. I deserve to be loved.
   - Children count. I do count.
   - I can give attention to my needs today.
   - Children are worthy. I am worthy of being with others.

8. Ask for a hug, a comforting hand, or to be held by someone you trust and someone who will ask nothing of you.

9. Acknowledge that you have taken action to move out of the pain. You are taking your life back.

Emotional Payoffs

You're continuing with a process that allows you to get your head and your heart working together. It has taken determination and guts to begin to incorporate the changes little by little into your life. You will recognize new freedoms and insights by conscientiously working the exercises and by allowing yourself time to process what the information means to you.

If you get stuck on an exercise, it may be more important to examine the reason why you're stuck than to complete it immediately. This healing process cannot be achieved simply by completing the written assignments as you would a school task, from A to Z. Your need to use food will gradually dissipate as you practice your new skills and become more confident.

In chapter 6, you're going to learn more about how to take control of your life and when to let go of control to ease your stress. Both aspects of understanding are essential in your eliminating food as a short-term fuel to gain a feeling of control. You'll learn to work more effectively with the only person who can control your life: You! You'll identify your life vision and eliminate destructive messages you load upon yourself and those messages shaped by family perceptions. You'll learn ways to achieve a balance between your desire to control and any tendency you have to assume responsibility for things over which you have absolutely no control.

Although we are focusing on the applications regarding your use of food, learning these tools will also continue to improve other elements of your life. Relationships at work and home can become more productive and enjoyable. Most important, your relationship with yourself will be free of all those old sabotages!

AFFIRMATION
Today I will meet my feelings head on,
accepting, listening, and honoring their purpose.

6

PRESCRIPTIONS TO PUT YOU IN CONTROL

Somewhere along the lines of development we discover what we really are, and then we make our real decision for which we are responsible. Make that decision primarily for yourself because you can never really live anyone else's life, not even your own child's. The influence you exact is through your own life and what you become yourself.

—Eleanor Roosevelt

Close your eyes and consider the freedom you would have if you took out all the shoulds, musts, and have-tos out of your life. Then, imagine everyone you are worried about taking care of their own problems.

What would you do with your time and energy?

Step 5: Know where to get control—and when to let it go.

Unfortunately, we can spend a good percentage of our time trying to control what we have absolutely no power to change. Because food issues are often born out of a need to gain control, knowing where to get control and when to let it go are crucial to focusing on your vision in life and reducing your reliance on food. As you have probably figured out, the more you rely on food for a feeling of control or power, the less you actually have.

If you have been frustrated because there never seems enough time to do or accomplish what you want, the following exercise will help you clarify where you are and what you need to do to change.

Achieving Your Life Vision: An Exercise

First, draw a circle or a box. Then, divide it into segments that represent the percentage of time you spend on family, work, spirituality, entertainment, exercise, health, self-help, and any other significant parts of your life.

Look at your completed exercise. If you continue allocating your time as you are, will you meet your life vision? Now create a second drawing, but change the percentage of each segment to reflect the balance you would like to attain.

Sometimes it's shocking to see how much time you spend doing things you do not want to do, or devoting time to things you cannot change or control. By viewing your time in this manner, you can see where it's possible to make small changes in your priorities to get you closer to where you want to be.

Start by thinking what you can control. For example, you may be spending more time than you'd like to at your job. Of course you can't quit your job, but you can limit how much time you spend on it. You can stop taking work or worry home. And, if you say that's not possible because your boss demands it, you can step back and see that you have three choices: remain in your job and establish boundaries on your time and workload; continue with the current workload and remain frustrated, but accept that you have made the choice to stay there and, therefore, don't have to overeat because you feel powerless; or you can recognize your frustration has been reasonable because work has been robbing you of personal time, and then begin preparing yourself to look for another job.

The nice thing about this vision is it is in your total control! You'll be surprised at how much better you'll feel with even small changes. One man became much more relaxed and serene just by eliminating a single daily ritual. Before he went to bed at night and first thing in the morning, he had been checking his business e-mail from home. There was no separation from work and personal time. When he decided to take a walk instead, he immediately felt more in control of his day. It also started on a more peaceful note.

Two more drawings will help further put you in control of your vision. Complete these drawings in the same manner as the previous exercise, but instead of activities, allocate your time currently spent in the following emotional states: joy, peace, worry, sadness, guilt, anxiety. Add any other emotion that takes up a lot of your time or that you think necessary for a satisfying life.

Now look at which emotional states you want to expand and which you want to decrease or delete. Then ask yourself, what do I need to do to make that happen? You're the only one who really has control. Begin with some type of change. It's as simple as that. Reflect upon your original drawings once a week. Make new ones and date them as you change. Continue for the next three to six months, building accountability for yourself and, equally important, accepting ownership for successfully taking control of the vision for your life.

If you find yourself reverting back to the "as-is" charts, stop and consider why. Are you losing yourself in other people's problems, problems that you really can't do anything about, or have no power to change? Parents and spouses are especially susceptible to this. For example, a mother can become extremely worried that a child is not going to pass a math class; she may pay for a tutor and spend an hour or two each evening working every math problem with (or for) the child. At every step, she pressures her child to pay attention. When the child gets to school and takes a test, she fails miserably because Mom isn't there to take it for her. Mom has assumed all the worry, and the child has taken no responsibility.

If Mom had set more reasonable boundaries, she could have let go of some of that worry and increased not only the possibility of her child passing math but also the possibility of improving their relationship. She could have told the child that, unless she studied at the kitchen table every night, there would be no TV—something Mom could control. She could not control whether the child tried to understand her math or not. Now the onus is on the child. She can ask for assistance, but Mom is no longer willing to take responsibility for her learning, other than providing reasonable help. The child learns there are consequences to her behavior. She'll be better equipped to cope with disappointments as she gets older, and her mother has more freedom to pursue her own life vision.

One of the most difficult times to admit your lack of control over another person is when a loved one is addicted to drugs or alcohol. It is difficult to move out of what you think is a helping role. But often, the more you "help" someone by making excuses for her behavior or bailing her out financially, the less that person has to be responsible for her own actions. She has no reason to stop the behavior. When you realize the only way you can help is by stopping your attempts to control the using, you put that person in a position to change and, finally, you have some release. When you've done everything you can do, such as getting a family intervention or counseling, you can be assured you've been a good parent or partner. That's why the Serenity Prayer, by Reinhold Niebuhr, is such an important tool in twelve-step programs. Consider how your life might change if you used this as a grounding tool each day:

God grant me the serenity
to accept the things I cannot change,
courage to change the things I can,
and wisdom to know the difference.

In your work thus far, you have shown a lot of courage to change things you can. There is a great deal of wrestling before we all realize the wisdom in knowing what we cannot change. You can't change your husband's annoying habits, or people from being abusive. However, you can change by telling them you will not participate in that abuse, you don't deserve it, and you won't absorb it. Then remove yourself from a destructive situation.

Its also helpful in a stressful situation to ask, Who am I turning the power *of my emotions* over to? At that point, you can do what you need to do to feel more in control. For example, at work you may be required to sit through an accusatory meeting that is rife with politics and personal agendas. However, you don't have to be pulled into others' chaotic spin. You can respond in a businesslike manner and know that, regardless of what happens in that meeting, you will still be the same, whole person when you leave. You have not given over control of your feelings or of the power to make you feel bad about yourself. Again, you have interrupted feelings that often lead to eating.

Changing Messages I Give Myself

You'd be surprised at how, by changing just your choice of words and the messages that you give yourself, you can put yourself more in control. Consider the following table. The messages in the first column make you feel incapable, shamed, trapped, or forced to do something. The messages in the second column put you in control. They also allow you to accept responsibility for the things you can change.

Restricting Messages	Empowering Choices
I don't have time	I'm choosing not to spend time on that.
I can't make a good grade in math.	I'm choosing not to try because there is a good chance I won't make better than a C, and that's not good enough for me.
I have to make a good impression.	I would like to make a good impression.
I should clean up the house.	I could clean house, but I'm choosing to give myself a goof-off day just for fun.
I must get into a top college.	I prefer to get into a top college, but I can get a worthwhile education elsewhere.

Changing your self-messages is a powerful move. Although part of your work is identifying where the old messages originated, it is equally important that you take responsibility for stopping them. Doing this work helps break the trigger to feelings of inadequacy, hopelessness, worthlessness, and other emotions that may have settled at your core.

You may be surprised at how often you give yourself self-destructive messages. Knowing just how often you do this can be overwhelming initially. However, it also firmly plants you in the driver's seat. If you know it, you can change it. Remember that each step in the Cycle of Pain reinforces the destructive use of food as a pattern to get out of the pain. When you take a chunk out of the cycle, it loses its momentum.

Begin today with some quiet thought. Ask, what messages do I give myself? Sometimes the messages you perceive from others today may become your own. For instance, if you think your husband believes you are undesirable because of your weight, you may internalize that message. If you believe a boss thinks you are inadequate, you may tell yourself, "I am stupid." Stacking up these negative messages will soon affect your confidence. Telling yourself "I am stupid" may soon make it difficult for you to do well on a test or to tackle a difficult situation for fear of failure. Or, you may spend a lifetime proving you are not stupid by engaging in a job that does not satisfy you. If you believe your negative messages, it will affect every aspect of how you live: your relationships, your job choices, and your parenting techniques. We'll continue to explore these messages, because they can be so destructive. You can obtain amazing freedom and control by identifying them, attacking them, and getting them out of your life.

For the next week, stop yourself when you give yourself a negative message. If you are flooded with them, a quick intervention is to just say no. This won't work long-term, but it may calm you long enough to take action on your feelings with reality checks or talkback, and after reflecting upon the purpose of the feeling, you can meet it head-on with other means to care for yourself, such as nurturing yourself when you are hurt or using affirmations to help boost your confidence. Using the following Ending Self-Destructive Negative Message Chart, write down the negative message and your response and then note how your feelings change when you take action. This exercise will give you areas to focus upon. Writing is another method to ground yourself and get out of overwhelming feelings.

During the second week, and as you progress further through the book, come back to this chart and identify additional ways you can talk to yourself, ways that will not engage you in the Cycle of Pain. Use the chart to connect with your feelings and to validate your ability to take positive actions for change.

The chart on page 78 provides examples of negative messages of the feelings they invoke, and of possible replacement messages. Read the examples, noting any similarities to your own messages. Then write down your own unique negative messages, and create some positive alternatives.

Changing Messages I Received from Others

The following exercise asks you to complete the statements you may have received from significant people in your life. It will help you identify why you may have bouts of overwhelming feelings. Although the form starts with messages from your mother, copy it and complete it again, substituting your father, spouse, and significant others.

Remember to also identify indirect messages, because they may be the ones that you internalized and that sabotage you today. Indirect messages may come in the form of avoidance, being ignored, being too busy, or not communicating positively with hugs, eye messages, or critical and disapproving looks. During this process, you will probably discover links to other core feelings.

For an example of an indirect message, consider a possible completion for sentence 11: "When I am critical of what you do ... I will raise my voice to tell you something must be wrong with you. Then I will not talk to you for a few days until I think you've learned your lesson." A child getting that message would feel ostracized for making mistakes or for making his mother unhappy. More than likely, he would develop a fear of making mistakes and either develop a driven

Ending Self-Destructive Negative Message Chart

Destructive Message	Feeling Afterward	Alternative Message	Feeling Afterward
I can't do anything right.	Hopeless, helpless, guilty, bad, less than, stupid, worthless	I need more information before I finish the project.	Hopeful, confident, focused
If only I tried harder, I could lose the weight.	Hopeless, guilty, bad, worthless, incompetent	I know now that losing weight is not a matter of willpower. I'm taking steps to feel better about myself and get to a healthy weight.	Hopeful, capable, directed, energized
If I weren't fat, my spouse/partner would show more affection.	Bad, less than, disgusting, guilty, numb, judged	My weight is only a part of who I am. My spouse/partner is using that as an excuse, instead of being honest and allowing us to work on problems in our relationship. He's not taking responsibility when he focuses only on my weight.	Free, a whole person, focused, worthy, equal

continued

Ending Self-Destructive Negative Message Chart

Destructive Message	Feeling Afterward	Alternative Message	Feeling Afterward
I'm bad because I can't stay on a diet.	Bad, disgusting, guilty, hopeless, not good enough, shameful, dissociated	Diets are uncomfortable and sometimes impossible to live with. I'm learning they are only a small part of the picture in weight issues. My eating too many calories or fats does not make me a bad person.	Confident, in control, hopeful, focused, energized

desire toward perfection or an attitude that he can't do anything right and is, therefore, a failure.

If completing the list discourages you, stop for awhile. But please come back. The feelings you are validating by completing the sentences are feelings you have carried for years, feelings that have been triggering your eating. By identifying their significance, you begin to change them. Without this knowledge, you are unable to do that. Your action as you complete the list shows you are taking charge of your life and are unafraid to meet challenges.

Messages That Impact My Life

My mother gave me the message:

1. When you were born, I felt
2. You are like me because
3. You are like your father because
4. You disappoint me because
5. You can meet with my approval and acceptance when
6. You can make me happy by
7. What I most like about you is
8. What I dislike about you is
9. My philosophy of life is
10. My main advice to you is
11. When I am critical of you, I will do or say
12. When I am complimentary of you, I will do or say
13. What I think of your worth as a person is
14. My beliefs about spirituality are
15. When you are an adult, I think you will be
16. My opinion of men is
17. My opinion of women is
18. My opinion of children is
19. My opinion of sexuality is
20. My beliefs about marriage are
21. My beliefs about fidelity are

22. My opinion about trust is
23. Love to me means
24. If you rebel, I will
25. My advice about your career choices is
26. Dreams are
27. I think your capabilities are
28. I think you are incapable of
29. Lying is
30. If you lie, I will react by
31. Weakness is
32. If you listen to me and watch my behaviors, you will see that I use manipulation to
33. If you listen to me and watch my behaviors, you will see I use food to
34. If you listen to me and watch my behaviors, you will see I use drugs and alcohol to
35. Safety to me means
36. If you or I are sick, we should
37. I think your needs are
38. As for you being able to take care of yourself, I think
39. If you listen to me and watch my behaviors, you will see that I think touch is
40. If you listen to me and watch my behaviors, you will see that I think control is
41. If you are afraid, it means
42. If I show you I am afraid, it would
43. I show you my attitude about anger by
44. I show you my attitude about rage by
45. I show you my attitude about manipulation by
46. My epitaph for you would be

After you've answered these questions (whew!), ask yourself what a child of five would feel like when receiving those messages?

How would a child of twelve feel? How would a child of seventeen feel? How do you feel today when you receive those messages from others or from yourself?

Circle the messages—both encouraging and critical—that you play in your head today. Are there any you have integrated into your belief system? Begin to take the power away from the negative messages. Reinforce positive messages.

For further power, write a paragraph about how each message has affected your development, education, relationships, career, and spiritual life.

In the Three Wishes exercise that follow, you'll discover if you are still giving yourself messages that prevent you from reaching your goals.

Exercise: Three Wishes

Remember what it was like as a child when you pretended to have a magic wand and wanted to believe that, when you closed your eyes and waved the wand, your fantasies would come true? Sometimes, even as an adult, you may be wishing and waiting for other people or circumstances to change in order for you to be happy. In your mind, freedom for you to pursue your dreams or be successful is dependent upon the action of others.

That illusion puts the power of your life into the hands of someone else over whom you have no control. Once you identify what your wish is, you take it out of the fantasy realm and put more realistic expectations on the only person whose actions you have power over. You!

For example, you may be holding back from finishing your college degree because you're wishing your spouse would be more supportive. You can accept that your spouse may not be totally supportive of your returning to school, and still get a college degree. You can also learn more effective ways to communicate with him, ways to express specifically what you mean by supportive. It may surprise you to discover that he thought he was being supportive, but that he defines it differently. It also might take some negotiating about family chores for your life to be easier while you are in college. But even if he refuses to help more around the house, you can still get that degree if it's what you want to do. You'll feel less frustrated once you lay your cards on the table and start directly addressing problems. And finally, when you stop putting your life on hold because you're waiting for other people, you may discover there is something you need to give yourself. For example, the woman who used her husband as an excuse not to go back to college also needed to face her insecurity about performing after being out of school for so long. Once she threw away the smokescreen her wish provided, she could focus on decreasing that fear. She began by contacting the university and connecting with others her age who had returned to school.

Use the following Three Wishes exercise to assess what is holding you back. Write your wishes, then think about why you have made that wish so important. If you, as an adult, could have three wishes concerning your mother, what would they be? Repeat the process with other significant people in your life.

1.

2.

3.

When you've completed the exercise, ask yourself the following questions:

1. Am I frustrating myself by longing for something unattainable?

2. Am I trying to get these wishes met by others or by food?

3. Am I using these wishes as excuses because I am afraid or insecure?

4. If these wishes about others do not come true, who can I rely on?

If you've answered yes to the first two questions, you now have freedom to let go of a wish you could never attain and to decrease the potential of your continuing to eat out of frustration or hurt feelings. A yes to question three signals that you are masking your own fears by focusing on the actions of others you can't control. Knowing that, you can dig deeper to explore what those fears are anchored to, then confront the feeling with your knowledge of trauma bonds, reality checks, talkback, and affirmations. You can take apart self-destructive messages.

The answer to question 4 is easy: Who do you have to rely on if your wishes don't come true? Just look in the mirror. You've worked hard to take apart the power of negative messages and reinforce your strengths. Without the wishes, you are free to face whatever is in your way. By taking small steps to meet your goals, you're more likely to achieve success.

In chapter 7, you're going to explore how loss has affected your life and how it, too, can remain as a roadblock. What you've learned about self-control will prepare you for facing those life experiences over which, for the most part, you probably had little control. You'll be surprised at discovering how much impact these losses have had on your life. You'll learn how recognizing and grieving a loss can help ease the painful feelings that have been with you since the loss occurred.

As you've learned ways to recognize and respond to the purpose of your feelings, you've boosted your ability to protect yourself assertively without food. By taking on some difficult emotional tasks, you've stopped relinquishing control of your life to others and to the scales. Before you start the next chapter, take a moment to reflect upon your progress and to own the positive changes you have made for yourself.

AFFirmaTion
Today I'm enjoying taking care of my own needs
and giving others the freedom
to assume personal responsibility.

7

OWNING YOUR
HIDDEN LOSSES

Some of your grief you have cured, and lived to survive;
but what torments of pain have you endured that haven't yet arrived.

—Ralph Waldo Emerson

Loss is an elusive thing. It can creep up on you over the years, causing an ache long disconnected from its birthplace. Or, it can hit with the intensity of a hurricane, wreaking havoc, destroying homes, taking lives. You salvage what you can, rebuild your home, or move away. The TV crews go home, and the enduring human spirit has dealt with another loss. Or has it?

It is the essence of human beings to survive. Sometimes acknowledging feelings appears to be a threat to that survival. Then, as organisms of life, we often kick into the mode that is most effective to disconnect from those feelings.

Take an aspirin and all your pain will go away. It's okay to grieve when someone dies—just don't let it go on too long and don't expect anyone else to talk to you about it. You can't acknowledge pain; such behavior is not manly. You can't let your children know how hurt you are because you must protect them at all costs. When your career path is broken by corporate politics, just move on and don't look back. When you have a miscarriage, it is better not to talk about it; that would cause too much pain, and people would think you are looking for pity. Your weight is your fault; therefore, you have no right to complain because you can't find clothes you like, because you face job discrimination, or because you are judged for what someone else sees during the first ten seconds of your meeting.

These messages are faulty. Yet we take them to heart and wrestle with the aftereffects for years. Buried deep, the unaddressed emotions become a sabotaging part of the Cycle of Pain. Triggered, they plunge us into coping by the destructive use of food. It's ironic that food is an accepted method for grieving in society, yet society can be harsh in judging the sometime consequences of extra pounds.

Although we all suffer from loss, there really is very little discussion about loss beyond the immediate occurrences. There often is debate about whether something is significant enough to be labeled a loss. Although some losses are very obvious, others are not so concrete. Wounds to the soul are internalized, hidden in the depths of our hearts. They lie unacknowledged and forgotten, yet their existence and the unresolved emotions they produced mark the beginning of a trauma bond that can interrupt our life's progression.

Step 6: Own, and then let go of your losses.
We move through stages of each loss, regardless of whether it is the death of someone we love, the end of a career, or the loss of a dream. One of the best frameworks for loss was developed by Elisabeth Kubler-Ross, author of *On Death and Dying*. She describes the stages of denial, anger, bargaining, depression, and acceptance. You may also feel despair and out of control. If you remain stuck in denial, because acknowledgement of and grieving for the loss are deemed unacceptable, the other feelings of despair, anger, and being out of control tend to dominate and shadow your potential to reach a stable, serene place in your life.

Overlooked Losses
Sometimes you may not consider a situation a loss because you didn't recognize the potential feelings it might evoke over a period of time. Being bullied as a child or not being accepted because of your weight

can result in feeling a loss of safety, or a loss of feeling secure. Adoption, which is a happy event for adoptive parents, provides another example. While it's easy to recognize the birth parent's loss, it is often more difficult to relate to the child's loss as a result of being placed for adoption, because the child has grown up in a home of love.

Connie is an adopted child who eats when she feels alone in the world, but she doesn't know why. She wrestles with an intense fear of abandonment even though she is being raised in a loving, protective home. As a dating teenager, she is afraid to let herself get too close to anyone for fear he will leave her. The boys she does choose say all the things she wants to hear, but their behaviors don't match. They treat her badly, then leave. They are experts at making her believe that the breakup is her fault or that something is wrong with her. Connie has mistaken their control for security and love.

Connie, who was saddled with extra pounds when her hormones began to change, became painfully self-conscious and began to believe something must be wrong with her because she just could not gain control of the pounds. Internally, she equates her biological mother's placing her for adoption with abandonment. Her interpretation is to believe she is unlovable. Connie has already begun to develop the belief that people she loves will leave her. Therefore, she must be unworthy or not good enough. She also feels a sense of loss as she wonders about the birth family she will never know and the life she might have had, although she does not share this with her parents. Since poor eating habits are almost expected in teens, it was easy for her to try to push down those intense feelings with food or to forget them by "forgetting" to eat. Until Connie changes the direction of her life by recognizing and working through these losses, her thinking and beliefs about herself will affect her relationships, career choices, and future parenting.

You'll discover how an environment of loss can drive your emotions and actions behind the scene as you read the following story about Carrie.

Long-Ago Losses

Carrie grew up in a family in which many people died. She began to believe that she would lose everyone close to her. Eating or not eating became the one thing she believed she could control. She became an overprotective adult who feared the world would hurt her husband and children. Her life became restrictive and closed. Instead of eating when she felt anxious, she "forgot" to eat when her stress increased or when something triggered her core feelings of being unsafe, abandoned, and out of control. Carrie wouldn't admit it initially, but fear was an underlying theme in her life. She fought it constantly until she realized she needed to fully grieve those old losses and dismantle the resulting core feelings and messages. With that recognition as a starting point, she began to stop the continuing interference from past loss and to eliminate her need to use not eating for a false sense of control.

As you delve deeper into uncovering loss in your life, you may still want to discount your pain and hang onto the denial of emotions that sustained you through a difficult time. However, as you share Eli's story in the next section, you'll see how that thinking only reinforces those feelings you have tried to repress and ultimately sabotages any efforts to attain a healthy weight. Your ignoring the feelings didn't make them disappear; they've continued to churn inside you, triggering attempts for relief through food.

Connecting to Losses and Finding Freedom

Unless you acknowledge hidden or past losses, you have no idea why you continue to hurt or why the intensity of those buried feelings is so disruptive that they cause you to overreact or numb out. Eli, a thirty-two-year-old computer professional, is still caught in emotional conflict that began years ago because he won't own his feelings and also strongly believes time should heal all wounds, particularly for men.

Eli replied when questioned about how his grandfather's death affected him, "I dealt with it and moved on." He rubbed his eyes, still not acknowledging the tears that lie just below the surface. "He raised me and I loved him very much. It was hard to see him go through the pain of cancer. But I'm an adult and I move on. I have to. I can't let it continue to affect me."

Eli's weight gain began almost immediately after he discovered that his grandfather had cancer. As the disease progressed, Eli used food to push down his feelings of fear, anger, and ongoing loss. He believed that, if he let those feelings surface, he would not be able to be strong for his grandfather. The more the illness got out of control, the more Eli's eating followed suit. Thirty pounds later and three years after his grandfather's death, he is carrying not only the unspoken feelings about his grandfather, but also new losses connected to carrying extra pounds. Connecting to that hidden loss at its source is far more essential than any new diet for Eli. Without that connection, he will not be able to sustain a healthy weight. The loss will continue to recycle and surface as extra weight.

Like Eli and Carrie, you may also be far removed from an original source of pain. To prevent continuous relapses into food issues, you must acknowledge both loss and the resulting core feelings as the triggers to the trauma bond. Otherwise, anytime something happens to trigger the intense hidden feelings, your first instinct will be to revert to a coping mechanism that has helped keep those feelings hidden. For you, it may be food. Sometimes, even after being in recovery for years, reaching for food is the first instinct.

Recognizing that food is your coping instinct gives you ammunition to realize one of two things. Either you are overreacting to a trauma bond, or you may be in an unhealthful or threatening situation today. Your feelings are telling you to slow down and survey what is going on. It is time to connect your head and heart to make decisions. Disconnect the pathway to the stomach that prevents you from moving forward, but listen to those urgings as warning signs. Food alone will not medicate away the pain. Neither will eating, purging, shopping, or using another compulsive behavior as a substitute to taking proactive action on your feelings.

Loss Experiences

Take a moment to reflect on your life. Have you had any of the loss experiences on the following list, or others that may have implanted a link between food and the feelings that resulted from the loss? As you read the list, allow your mind to be open to exploration. Circle those that you've experienced. Jot down any thoughts related to each loss as you go, or you may forget them by the end of the list. Remember that dissociating or forgetting is a coping mechanism. And if you eat after looking at the list, and still think you are not affected by loss, think again. The list may hold clues for you to end that constant battle with weight.

Exercise: Identifying Your Losses

1. Death of a parent, child, sibling, grandparent, other relative, or person who had significance in your life
2. Suicide of a relative, friend or classmate
3. Living (or lived) in an alcoholic home or a home with a parent who had an untreated emotional problem
4. Serious medical problem, one time or chronic
5. Involved in an accident
6. Physical abuse
7. Sexual abuse
8. Emotional battering or controlling
9. Natural disasters
10. Close calls with your life or someone's life who is important to you
11. Divorce of your parents or divorce from your spouse
12. Child of a parent who left or who did not maintain close contact after divorce
13. Placing a child for adoption
14. Miscarriage
15. Stillborn child
16. Being adopted

17. Being teased or bullied as a child or teen
18. Being an outcast or perceiving yourself as one
19. Living in a fishbowl because of your parents' public jobs, such as pastor, therapist, politician
20. Loss of privacy due to parental overinvolvement or boundary violations by others
21. Financial devastation
22. Disillusionment or disappointment with life
23. Disillusionment or disappointment with marriage
24. Betrayal or hurt by someone you trusted, or should have been able to trust
25. Infertility
26. Loss of identity
27. Loss of freedom
28. Feelings of inferiority because of your weight (it doesn't matter if you perceived you were underweight or overweight)
29. Lack of attention from parents
30. Attention Deficit Disorder
31. Learning disabilities
32. Significant problems in your children despite your attempts to be a healthy parent
33. Loss of a dream
34. A violent home
35. Loss of a family illusion
36. Having a child who has emotional or addiction problems
37. Loss of a playful, safe childhood
38. Role reversals that placed you in a position of trying to fulfill a more adult role as a child
39. Loss of innocence
40. Loss of life as it should be
41. Foster care
42. Other losses :

How do you feel after reading this list: overwhelmed, sad, numb, out of touch, fearful? Watch your reactions during the next eight hours. Remember, if you find yourself reaching inappropriately for food, the list probably set off a core feeling. Recognizing that connection is the first step in making it go away. Since you have validated your feeling instead of running away, you can begin to search for the feeling's purpose and take affirming action by using grounding techniques or talkback, by attacking any self-destructive messages—in short, by using all the tools you learned in earlier chapters.

You may say that everyone has these things happen at some time. It's not necessarily true, and if it were true, it would not matter. Your loss is real. It hurts. It affects you in many ways. Just acknowledging this fact aloud can be a powerful first step in decreasing its impact on your weight issues. Having a stiff upper lip and going on can be quite helpful at times. But a stoic facade eventually collapses inward, like the implosion of a building. Implosion protects the environment, but the building is demolished. That is what happens to people. When the rubble is cleared away, the ghosts remain.

Even when one has worked through emotional residue, there still remains the loss of what was or what could have been. But if you have done effective work, the loss no longer continuously sabotages you. Of course, nothing really ever makes a loss totally disappear. It may crop up with a memory. Your object is not to erase it, only to acknowledge it. If it does crop up, let yourself listen, feel, and acknowledge that it was a painful time. It is sad to have lost someone or something important to you. But it is dangerous to link that sadness to a lifetime of guilt, rejection, loneliness, or powerlessness.

Unrecognized Losses

As you review your losses, use the following chart to determine how they may have affected your life. When connections are repressed, it's sometimes most effective to assume the role of the objective reporter. In the first column, identify the losses you have had. Jot down the facts, as if you were an impartial observer. Ask yourself the reporter's standard questions: who, what, when, where, and why? Who did the loss occur to and who was involved? What happened? When and where did it happen? And finally, why did it happen? Of all those questions, you will find the last question the most difficult one to answer, and often it may not even be possible. Focusing too long on the why in this case may create despair and hopelessness. For now, focus more on the facts you know.

Next, in the second column, write down what you felt as you gathered the information in column one and what you may have felt during the original experience. If it is difficult for you to identify feelings because you have blocked them in the past, imagine again you're the reporter, writing down the feelings someone else might have had during such an event. You may have more empathy for others than for yourself. List these feelings.

In the third column, go one step further and begin to brainstorm about how those feelings may have affected you (or that other person). How could it have affected you (or the other person) developmentally? What would be its effect on relationships, school performance, careers, choices?

Use the information you have gathered as a road map to set your plan of action. Now that you recognize the far-reaching impact the loss has made in your life, use the knowledge you gained in chapter 3

Loss Connections		
Loss	Possible Hidden Core Feelings	How That Loss Affected My Life

about disconnecting from trauma bonds to begin to break free. Search for core feelings, be on the lookout for feelings flashbacks, and look for core messages that are connected with your loss. Use the techniques you've learned about validating your feelings and replacing negative messages to attack and dismantle the negative consequences of unrecognized loss. You'll find that, in accepting the loss, you have given yourself permission to let it go.

Specific Losses

In the next sections, we'll take an in-depth look at some of the most frequently overlooked losses. As you read the stories, underline what is similar to your experiences or feelings. Think specifically about what personal assets you have used to pull yourself through these or similar difficult times. Jot them down and attach them to your Loss Connection Chart so that you will be able to keep in mind your strengths. Your life will only get richer by the work you are doing.

You also will identify core feelings and messages as you relate to the loss experiences. Remember that the ongoing identification of core feelings and messages is a crucial part of your work, work that ultimately will make this experience at ending weight issues different from those efforts you have previously made.

Take your time and don't rush through the remainder of this chapter. You may be making connections to areas of loss you had not considered or had pushed aside. It's time to roll up your sleeves for some of that emotional sweat that I promised. Keep in mind that the process will help you make sense of your life and will help you lose the emotional weight that is holding you back.

Family Illusion: Abuse in the Home

If you were a child in a home when sexual abuse, physical threats, or violence occurred, you may literally have feared for your life. If you did not accept the world as presented to you, that danger may have actually increased. How could anyone predict when an out-of-control adult would take it one step further?

Destructive words, particularly by people you love, also can affect your development and relationships well into adulthood. You no doubt will suffer the consequences when you are told that you are not good enough, that you have to try harder, that something is wrong with you, or that you should never have been born. It is an incredible loss not to be able to approach life with the feeling that you are wanted or that you are a whole person.

With abuse comes the loss of safety, of privacy, and of setting our own boundaries. Control is taken away. We lose freedom, choices, and often identity because we believe we must be chameleons to accommodate and survive the abusers' moods. The abuse may have been just a threat, may have occurred once, or may have occurred hundreds of times. Nonetheless, the wounds are deep.

In a troubled environment, sometimes illusion is all that holds you together. Sometimes this illusion is fed by an active imagination. Other times it is reinforced by feelings of appropriate closeness or love that exist in areas away from the abuse. Even abusive or dysfunctional families may have moments of healthier interactions, closeness, or laughter. Thus, the family illusion becomes stability, and reality only an illusion. And one of the illusions is that it is much easier to accept responsibility for everything that goes wrong than to believe that people who are supposed to love and take care of you are hurting you or others. That is how core feelings of being bad, responsible, guilty, and powerless evolve. Core messages might include: "I can't do anything right." "There must be something wrong with me." " I'm stupid." "I must be worthless." "Life is hopeless." "I am powerless, frozen, trapped." "People in authority can hurt me." "Love and abuse go together." "If people knew the real me, they would leave me." "I have to dissociate, or ignore reality in some way to avoid the pain and survive." "I cannot control myself." (That core message may be one that you beat yourself up regularly with as it relates to food.) "I must be in control to be safe."

Those thoughts and feelings are overwhelming, prompting you to begin to use food to dissociate or prompting you to become numb during troubled times. It is safer to go someplace else in your mind than to confront your fears. You can also begin eating to soothe anxiety, to push down rage or anger, to rebel and to gain control. Remember, you have already learned to decrease the power of trauma bonds that enact those same core feelings and messages today by recognizing triggers and stopping feelings flashbacks. You have done this with grounding techniques and reality checks, then talking back and replacing the trauma- or loss-based core messages with more positive, realistic ways to think about yourself and the situation. Thus, you have circumvented the need for your old destructive coping mechanisms. By acknowledging the loss, you have reached an advanced level in this healing process.

You don't have to live with the legacy of that abuse. Knowledge gives you power to break what may have been a pattern for several generations in your family. The changes that you are making can have an uplifting impact on you, your significant others, your children, and even generations to come.

Strengths as an Abuse Survivor

If you were from a troubled family, you have had to exhibit inordinate strength and wisdom to survive. You have had to be creative to get out of tough situations. You've had to depend upon your ability to think through problems. All these are powerful assets in your quest to end your struggles with your weight and to gain acceptance of yourself.

As you read and complete the exercises in this book and continue to put together the pieces of your unique puzzle, you'll be able to use this wisdom and ability to assess situations with open eyes and to make those important connections that will help you bring about positive change. You've already increased your coping and problem-solving skills. And finally, when you begin to recognize your inner strength, you will be more secure in life and more at peace with yourself. You'll find, with that confidence, that there will be fewer struggles—not only where food is concerned but also in personal relationships and life choices.

Pushed to Perfection

Sometimes even well-meaning parents hurt their children. In their quest to protect and prepare them for the future, they overdo. They push and push. Ironically, sometimes these parents were hurt themselves. In their quest to provide their children with a safer environment and more opportunities, they load up the restrictions and pressures. They also tend to take too much responsibility for their children's behavior and emotions. Although done in love and a sense of protection, this behavior robs you of your capacity to own your emotions and use them to problem-solve, to feel that you are capable and able to handle disappointments. You can grow up thinking that making a mistake makes you a failure, instead of viewing a mistake as a natural part of your learning experience. Your parents' best intentions can actually teach you to shirk responsibility, the exact opposite of their goals.

You may also naturally be a more sensitive person, one who overreacts to the opinions of others and who may have perceived more pressure than your parents intended. If your parents have jobs that put them in the public eye, such as a politician, pastor, teacher, or therapist, you may have perceived that you had to live up to a higher standard than others. Thus, you may have begun a lifelong pattern of being a perfectionist, expecting unrealistically high standards of others, of yourself, and even of your own body.

Death of a Child

The death of a child is one of the most painful and difficult losses to bear. If you have lost a child, you know the stress is crushing. The divorce rate is extremely high for parents who have suffered a child's death. Guilt, anger, and a mixture of other emotions are officially buried with your lost child, yet these feelings may linger for years.

As one woman explained, while wiping away tears, "I tried so hard to make everything perfect for her—normal." The fifty-year-old woman was speaking of her little girl, who died at the age of seven, more than twenty years ago. Maggie had been diagnosed with major health problems as an infant, and each day had been a gift. However, years of living on borrowed time wore down her mother and father. Her mother disclosed, "When she died, of course everything wasn't normal. I blamed myself because I had not found the treatment that would have worked for her to get better. If I had just tried harder, maybe I could have saved her life. I cried and cried. Finally my husband and his family pressured me to get hold of myself and go on. I had other kids, too. But the pain never went away." The tears continued. "No one listened. No one cared. I felt so alone."

Her weight problems began with her daughter's illness and increased substantially after her death. Her husband, in his need to fix something, began to focus on his wife's weight. He could not control the illness that stole his daughter, so he turned his out-of-control feelings onto his wife, constantly pressuring her to exercise, eat less, and look better. Instead of talking about his pain, he became angry. He blamed her weight for problems in their marriage. But most of the problems in their marriage came from the crushing pain of losing a child and from not knowing how to grieve through the hurt.

The core feelings that evolved for both parents were similar, yet their grief isolated them. If they had talked about their feelings, they could have supported each other through this loss. Maggie's illness and death initiated their feelings of terror that they might lose her, of lack of control, and of hopelessness, of rage at having their child taken from them, and of despair at never being able to see her enjoy the dreams they had for her. They lost so much. Yet they were not able to talk about it at all.

Miscarriages and the birth of a stillborn child are other significant losses often shuffled out of sight. The mother's feelings are often particularly undervalued; she is supposed to, but of course is unable to, take comfort from misguided comments such as "It was for the best" or "It's a good thing you didn't get attached." But, while the pain is every bit as real as for an older child, it is often more difficult to work through, because experiences with this baby were not long-term. In order not to use food or other medication to fill the emptiness and to get through the loss, you must acknowledge it is normal for you to have intense pain with a miscarriage and to honor the lost baby's existence and your grief over the baby's death.

Choosing to let go of your grief is difficult, but it is vital. Grief does not disappear with the passage of time, by ignoring it, or by numbing out your feelings with food. You'll have to make a conscientious choice to acknowledge the loss and the feelings surrounding the loss before you are able to release its grip and establish some serenity. For some it feels as if grief is the only connection to the lost child. However, as you begin to acknowledge your grief and let it go, you will see it allows you to integrate your child's memory in a way that is much richer, and you will find that you will be able to honor your lost child as a part of you.

Death of Other Family Members

We often underestimate the effect of a family member's death, particularly upon a child, because children are often unable to express themselves or even to be in touch with their loss. Parents may be so lost in their own grief that they are relieved to see their children return to their activities so quickly, wanting to believe that the children are only mildly affected. Yet, this activity may be the children's way of running from the pain, from the emptiness they feel. As a consequence, this avoidance may set the pattern for a desire to run, or to eat to fill the emptiness whenever you feel threatened with loss later in life.

As Eli's case showed, adults also can begin to have eating problems around the time of a life-threatening chronic illness or a death. It is acceptable to find solace in food during those times. Yet months later when a life event that once would have been shared with your loved one triggers that raw feeling of loss again, no one, including yourself, is too forgiving of your bingeing. Writing a letter to the person who died sometimes helps ease the pain but will not take away the loss. It can, however, take away the immediate need to reach for food to fill an emptiness that can't be filled. You know from your reading in previous chapters that, by taking action, you have begun to ground yourself and move out of the past to the present, where you can do something effective with your feelings.

The suicide of a friend or loved one takes emotional hostages. Because it is often not talked about, even among family members, the loss becomes twisted and tangled. Guilt and often-repressed anger shadow a healthy recovery. But your life does not have to be directed by the action of someone over whom you really had no control. As James recounted, "I avoided conflict my whole life." His father committed suicide when James was sixteen. "I missed opportunities and let myself get stepped on. It wasn't because I was chicken, not at all. I was afraid of what would happen if I let my anger get out. I knew it was powerful and I might be sorry. So I always walked away. Over the course of years, I lost a lot of self-respect. I began to feel like a failure.

"I drank a lot after my dad's death. Then when I figured out I couldn't get through school unless I stopped, I guess I moved on to food. I never realized until recently that the anger I was afraid of had been churning inside me all these years. I was so angry at my dad for leaving me, I couldn't stand it. I was afraid if I said anything to anyone, I would sound disloyal. I loved him. But he betrayed me by leaving that way.

"I was just like a kid in an abusive family. I would rather bury my anger with food than acknowledge that someone I loved so much had hurt me, and I was incredibly angry because of it. My anger directed me. It restricted me. When I got the courage to look at it and voice it, I felt incredible relief. My life started making sense and I felt I had more control.

"I still love my dad, but I don't have him on a pedestal anymore." He shook his head. "That pedestal was killing me."

If someone you know has committed suicide, you know feelings of anger, guilt, and lack of control often dictated your thoughts related to that person in the past. Validating and acting upon those feelings can provide freedom. You are taking active steps to honor the loss and recognize the person as a human being who made a devastating choice, not as a superhero. Knowing you can still love a person whose actions hurt you allows you to let go of the unreasonable guilt and anger you held onto, fearing that acknowledging it would lessen that love. Anyone can see that James's father's suicide was beyond his control, just as most of our losses in life are.

You have learned that there is no shame in owning a vast array of feelings after a loss. Time does not heal all wounds, but the validation of your pain and the work you are doing can.

Infertility

Infertility is packed with many losses: the loss of parenthood, the loss of a normal relationship as all attention is focused on the drive to become pregnant, financial losses from the expense of fertility treatments. Couples accept these losses as they wage a private war to beat their own bodies.

If you do not have a successful pregnancy, losses continue because you have no child to focus on. But grieving the inability to conceive is often neglected. Even if you successfully give birth, the pain of those months never goes away, nor does the fear that it will happen again if you try to have a second child. This fact places quite a bit of pressure on you and your child.

Gretta began, "Everything in our lives was focused on my getting pregnant." She shook her head. "There was absolutely no romance to our sex because it was timed and focused on demand. I submitted to every medical procedure conceivable. I was obsessed. When I finally did get pregnant, I was overwhelmed with the feeling that I would lose this baby. After the baby was born, I acted as if that feeling had never happened. But I noticed I already had starting gaining weight long before the pregnancy. I needed something to fill my emptiness."

Gretta's fear of losing the baby continued to affect her as the child grew up. She became so overprotective that, by the daughter's teenage years, the child still had not learned how to handle disappointment. Gretta and her husband treated her differently, because she was "special" and the product of so many losses. As a result, the daughter didn't have to be accountable for her mistakes. Family counseling helped them sort through these effects.

When you suffer through a loss such as infertility, it is important to take pride in your strengths in getting through trying times. You are willing to try new tactics to solve problems. You can focus on a goal during stressful times. You have shown remarkable stamina, because month after month, you persisted when your hopes had gone unrewarded. These strengths and stamina are assets in many areas of your life; all will help you to address both this loss and the other issues around food and weight.

Abortion

Abortion is never an easy decision. Most women make it when they feel they have no other choice. Those who believe they are aborting a baby face the same excruciating pain and loss as anyone who loses a child. If you feel that way, it is important to go through a focused grieving process for that baby, giving it a name and honoring it. For others, abortion remains a loss of control and perhaps a loss of their ideal of pregnancy. Women may fear it will hamper future pregnancies. It may mean the loss of a relationship. Core feelings include guilt, fear, or being trapped, abandoned, or betrayed. Core messages can include the following: "I can't do anything right." "I made the choice; therefore, I can't complain of any pain." "I am bad."

As you begin to relate to any core feelings or messages, acknowledge that you were in a difficult situation. Envision for a moment the environment and circumstance that led you to your decision. They were probably extremely stressful. Forgive yourself. You did the best you could. Isn't it time to stop hurting yourself and let go of the pain? Sometimes we become our most critical judges.

Adoption

If you have ever placed a child for adoption, you know it is an anguishing decision, and it is a gift of ultimate love that few can come close to understanding. You may have had other people judging you, but you are hurt more if you beat yourself up for a decision made during a time in your life when probably there were few choices. Women in therapy after placing their child often exhibit gut-wrenching grief. Many refuse to address it in a healthful way for fear they will not be able to hang on to sanity. Meg expressed this fear and grief: "If I let myself think of my little baby for even a moment, I'd get so depressed. Frozen. I couldn't work. I couldn't get out of bed. I know I made the right decision for her, because I couldn't raise a child at that time. There are people out there who think I did something unthinkable, yet I did it out of love."

Placing her child for adoption evoked core feelings of guilt, worthlessness, despair, loneliness, and loss of control. She also felt trapped because she had no other choice and because she felt that she had betrayed her child, even though rationally she knew she was making the best choice for both her and the baby. The strongest core message that followed for Meg was "I am bad."

Meg began to miss meals and ignore her body's messages of hunger. As you'll learn more about in chapter 9, restricting food can actually give some people a power surge. At a point in her life where Meg felt she had little control over anything, she was making a statement that she could control what she ate or didn't eat. She received not only the initial chemical reaction within her body, a reaction that felt good, but an additional payoff in recognition from others that she had lost weight. Yet, once she started this path, she found it difficult to stop and did not start eating healthfully again until a concerned and loving girlfriend confronted her. It took some-one on the outside to jolt Meg back to reality by calling attention to how she was hurting herself: she was losing too much weight and get-ting physical complications; she was having trouble concentrating; she had increasing problems at work; she became isolated from her friends and was always unhappy. Meg said, "I had to talk about what I was feeling to survive. I was only fooling myself by thinking I could rid myself of those strong emotions by not eating. I just kept hurting myself, and I guess in a way I felt I deserved it. When I recognized I was making all my decisions based on giving myself that core message 'I am bad,' I realized I would never get out of despair unless I took charge of my life. I started by owning how I felt about giving up the baby, then using what I have learned to attack the garbage messages I kept loading on myself. I can't tell you how much relief I feel today.

"I haven't forgotten my baby. I've just chosen to put her in a spe-cial place in my heart that's filled with love now, instead of with those horrible feelings of despair and guilt."

If you are an adopted child, you also may suffer from a wounded soul. Although you may have had no physical memory, you can carry core feelings of being abandoned, worthless, and lonely. The result-ing core messages include these: "I'm bad." "Something must be wrong with me or I wouldn't have been placed for adoption." "I'm unlovable." "People who I love will leave me." These feelings often erupt more strongly during preteen and adolescent years, and may cause considerable disruption. These years are also a time that you are more vulnerable to weight gain, both because of hormonal changes and a normal teenager's junk eating habits.

Adoptive parents should discuss with their child the loss of birth parents, just as you would discuss the death of a family member. The child lost a crucial connection when he or she was placed for adop-tion. To consider the connection nonexistent because we replace the family is negating the depths of the human soul. The loss is real for both the birth mother and the adopted child. Feelings of abandonment and of not being worthwhile, fears of rejection and of not wanting to hurt anyone can be extreme. Connecting to these feelings at the source with the tools you have learned is a way to validate them.

While this idea may seem complex, the most powerful force motivating those involved in adoption is the circle of love. Recognizing this loving support can provide a base for any work you may have in this area, whether you are the birth parent or the adopted child. With the completion of Step 6 and with your awareness of the impact of this loss, you can then use your knowledge of breaking trauma bonds, connecting your use of food to your feelings, and attacking garbage messages to bring a new acceptance of your whole self into everyday life choices. You'll find you have increased substantially your confidence and ability to make changes.

Foster Care

Children placed into foster care often grow up with a combination of core feelings and messages, not the least of which are abandonment, and feeling unlovable and worthless. If you were a foster child, you may have suffered from many of the losses discussed in this chapter. Don't become overwhelmed. The work you do on one loss will help you validate and let go of the others.

It takes quite a bit of perseverance and guts to weather a foster care system. You probably have learned to problem-solve in difficult circumstances. You have learned to depend upon yourself. You may even have developed a sense of stubbornness, which you can turn into positive persistence today as you work to let go of your losses. Finally, instead of having to use all those strengths for survival, you can use them to enrich your life.

Divorce

Although in our overly civilized society we like to think that people can successfully move past a divorce, we cannot negate losses: loss of love, loss of dreams, and often loss of financial stability.

Core feelings may include betrayal, fear, or loneliness, and you may feel repulsive, unlovable, undeserving, and trapped. The following core messages may be activated: "I must be a failure. I can't do anything right." "There must be something wrong with me." "If he (or she) doesn't love me, no one else can." "I will be alone forever." "It's not safe to allow myself to love anyone. I cannot afford to be vulnerable again."

Children often feel the same way. You can become extremely harmed when your noncustodial parent walks away and has no consistent contact—even if it occurs before you are old enough to talk. You can grow up with a legacy of rejection. This legacy also can happen if your parents were not married and one leaves. As Carmen, a fifty-year-old professional woman, disclosed, "I never knew it, but for years my relationships were attached in an odd way to my father's leaving. I never really let myself get close to a man for fear he would leave me. The guys I chose were guys who seemed real secure and sure of themselves. But they were really just controlling. I separated from and returned to my husband four times before I finally left him. By that time he had hurt me terribly. There were other women. He was spending all our money. And I'm the one that felt terrible. I was afraid of hurting him.

"I would sneak food and eat after we had fights or after I found another note from one of his girlfriends. Then he would constantly berate me about my weight. I finally figured out that I did not want to lose any weight because then he would win. I didn't want to give in to him one more time. My weight was my stand. He really could not control it.

"I know I paid a bunch of consequences for that thinking. I felt really bad about myself. But my little island of power was my weight. When I figured out why I was doing it, I started looking at the deeper reasons I was attracted to him and stayed with him in the first place. In some way I was equating my leaving him with my father leaving me. Through the years I just did not want anyone else to feel the same incredible hurt of being abandoned and rejected. I couldn't stand feeling responsible. I didn't want to be like my dad. I knew how bad I felt as a child, wondering what was so wrong with me that he could just disappear and pretend I didn't exist. But really, my father leaving did not have anything to do with me being good or bad. It had to do with his decision as an adult."

With that recognition, it did not take Carmen long to stop using food destructively. As she discarded old pain, she found she became more confident and assertive in meeting her needs. When she felt controlled, she talked about it. Food, she realized, had lost its effectiveness. She also found she was no longer willing to be in relationships with men who were not emotionally available for her, and she was able to leave with no guilt.

Accidents, Injury, Illness, and Other Close Calls

There are times that jar us out of the ordinary. We can no longer experience life in the same way because of circumstances that disable us or bring us close to death. The losses are immediate and shocking, whether we are the victims or someone we care about is hurt. We can no longer naively go through life as if it will never end. Though for a brief time after physical recovery, we may treat life even more preciously, eventually we step back on the treadmill of work and too many responsibilities.

These journeys into uncertainty, however brief, signify loss in many ways. There may be physical aftereffects. We may never again regain our strength or capabilities. Or, there may be emotional problems. We can be left with the lingering fear that it will happen again, and the next time it could take even more from us.

One woman in recovery for food issues began bingeing and compulsively shopping after her young son was hit by a car. Miraculously, he escaped with only minor injuries. She experienced great relief. But that still did not negate the overwhelming fear and shock she felt when the realization sank in of how close she came to losing him.

Speaking of the accident, she said, "I felt so much terror, so out of control. I ate steadily for a week. I knew what I was doing, though, and it concerned me.

"I had fought long and hard for this recovery and I wasn't going to throw it away," she said with clenched fists. "I had used food to get me through those first days. Then I realized it was time for me to talk about what I was feeling. I knew the food wasn't going to work for me, and I was worried that if I didn't do something, I would lose control."

"If I had not learned how to stop core feelings and despair from taking over, I would have started purging again. I had learned through my reading that I was experiencing a normal reaction to a traumatic event, but I also realized I was not doing what I needed to do to keep it from haunting me and sending me right back to food. I was not talking about it, I wasn't even letting myself feel. I knew I was in a serious situation and I had to do something about it. I called my therapist, because this time it was just too big for me to handle alone."

It took only a few sessions for her to stop the binge cycle. She used a combination of the tools you have learned plus a fierce determination not to let herself go backward. She began by noting all the different feelings she was experiencing, by accepting that it was realistic to experience these feelings because her son's accident was a traumatic loss, and by recognizing that she could not always keep him safe. She then used the grounding techniques she had learned to stop these feelings from continuously flooding her and to determine whether the accident had prompted the re-emergence of trauma bonds tied to the past. With that knowledge, she was able to address those feelings quickly and pay full attention to her immediate needs. She concluded, "Just by acknowledging I was in the middle of a traumatic experience and being able to give names to what I was experiencing, I regained some sense of control and direction. Instead of it pushing me into further chaos, I stepped up my nurturing of myself as well as the nurturing of my son. When I saw I was beginning to dissociate, I knew to pull back. I was happy, too, that I could use reality checks and assertiveness confidently as tools to help my son get through the health care system."

Using the knowledge she had learned, she faced a situation that would be traumatic to anyone and gained recognition that what she had learned had now become a part of her. She quickly sought out healthy ways to meet her needs. That same confidence will build with you as you continue to let go of your loss. You'll soon find that by acknowledging your complete range of feelings and practicing techniques you now know will help you address your needs, you'll be more in control, more directed and less likely to use food in an attempt to push down feelings.

Letting Go Brings Peace

Now that you have owned your losses by accepting their consequences and your resulting feelings, you have started to break the Cycle of Pain. Acknowledging the loss won't make you feel worse; it will allow you to release pain you have been carrying around. Unrecognized, the pain roars inside you like a tornado, causing disruption without your knowing how to stop it. Since you now understand the pain and the actions you have blindly taken in the past to push it down, the pain has begun to dissipate.

In the next chapter, you'll enter the final stage of working through emotional connections to food. You'll learn additional ways to let go of the natural feelings of anger that accompany any loss. The techniques you'll gain will be useful to finish up the work you have already completed on trauma bonds and to feel freedom from the past. You'll also be experiencing ways that you can face your anger on a daily basis, and you can take steps to address it when it happens—rather than letting it build.

Today you are no longer handcuffed to an invisible loss. By acknowledging that the loss was real and your hurt was a normal reaction, you have moved forward and broken out of the Cycle of Pain. Your willingness to examine even the most painful parts of your life to discover solutions demonstrates even more clearly your strong inner drive to find answers. That underlying courage will continue to blossom not only as you progress through this book but as you practice your new coping skills and celebrate more and more the strengths you have.

AFFIRMATION
Today I will allow myself to fully experience life
by setting free my pain
and honoring my losses
with a special place in my heart.

8

Make Anger Work For You

Anyone can become angry—that is easy. But to be angry with the right person, to the right degree, at the right time, for the right purpose, and in the right way—this is not easy.

—Aristotle

If you have had a lifetime of struggles with your weight, you are probably struggling with a sleeping volcano—anger. It constantly bubbles and churns below the surface until eventually it erupts. The fire then spurts forth uncontrollably, and everyone around you— from your boss to your children—can become victims. Or the eruption drives inward, turning into a powerful depression. You can suffer it quietly by eating the anger, by controlling your fear or disgust of the anger, or by swallowing the emotion. The volcano represents years of repressed feelings: hurt, frustration, fear, shock, and anger. If you are hurt as a child, you can drag into adulthood a legacy of fear that cripples the expression of your true feelings. You are trapped with a programmed belief that validation of these feelings will spark intense physical or emotional pain, perhaps even cause loss of family. It becomes far easier to push them down by manipulating them with food.

One roadblock to acknowledging anger is the reluctance to cast blame on others. But acknowledging anger is not placing the responsibility of your life in someone else's hand. It is about making others accountable for their behavior and identifying its effects on you. When that recognition occurs, you can free yourself from undeserved guilt and can decrease the tendency of guilt and anger to trigger destructive eating.

You may fear that you will lose your relationship if you acknowledge the truth, but that rarely happens. More likely, it will change for the better: you'll be more comfortable with yourself, and you'll have an opportunity to have a more meaningful relationship. Remember that you have already successfully completed steps that also confront the past. You're totally in the driver's seat as you continue to explore how you can further make your feelings work for you today, instead of letting those feelings drive you to food.

Step 7: Make anger work for you: Identify how your ideas about anger and rage were shaped by your environment growing up, and learn more effective ways to express yourself today.

Looking at the purpose of any feeling makes it easier to understand. Anger is a healthy emotion, designed to protect us. It serves as a warning signal. If you are angry, it means you are being hurt emotionally or physically and you need to step back to assess the situation. If you are in danger, leave. In other instances, using what you have learned about being assertive can help you take care of yourself without hurting others.

Your family may have pretended they were never angry. If so, you were denied a valuable experience of watching how anger can protect you and be used to move toward solutions to problems or away from danger.

Anger vs. Rage

Maybe you may have had a family where rage—not anger—was the norm. If you grew up in a troubled home, you can have a difficult time in distinguishing rage from anger. If your family screamed, hit, threw things, or threatened you or other family members, you were in an environment of rage. You may have become more confused if the person raging later apologized for "my anger."

In its purest form, rage is a raw release of emotion that occurs in response to something that is beyond comprehension. For example, rage occurs when someone intentionally hurts another, particularly a child; rape generates rage. Rage also can occur when you suffer any significant loss, such as the death of a loved one or a chronic illness. If you acknowledge the feeling at that time, you may react with a raw, primal scream or your body may literally shake in its devastation. You may cry uncontrollably. If those expressions of rage can be connected to an event, you can experience a tremendous amount of release. Rage allows you to let go and move forward because rage in its healthy use triggers an emotional release of pain and suffering. Once you acknowledge you have a right to the initial rage you feel, then you can move to anger, where you can take action. Remember, rage is to release emotions, and anger promotes further action to protect.

Rage also can become a dissociative state. It is often triggered by other core feelings, and it can provide an immediate sensation of power. However, rage can become a very out-of-control feeling where violence of hands, words, or actions erupts. It is often used as an excuse to hurt, either physically or with the cold, calculated silence that signifies judgment or withdrawal of love. For example, one woman remembered as a child being afraid to speak up for herself or talk to her brother after her father refused to speak to her twelve-year-old brother for six weeks. Her brother's crime was asking why his father did not like one of his friends. Another young woman, who initially was unable to identify a threatening environment, remembered her father's judgmental stares and occasional hitting the walls with his fists. The threat was implied.

Later in the chapter, you'll learn more about the difference between rage and anger and become more comfortable with the healthy, protective uses of anger.

Breaking the Ties to Food

Without the knowledge of how to express anger safely and beneficially, your anger can fester for years—often without your knowing it.

You may reach for food to soothe those totally unacceptable feelings. Or, in an act of violence against your body, you may purge through vomiting, laxatives, compulsive eating, or exercise. Maybe you're an anorexic who turns rage inside by restricting food. This dangerous, symbolic flirting with death is perceived by some as the ultimate expression of rage. Take the example of Frank.

Frank was in therapy for his weight problems for three months before he had any memories of the first eighteen years of his life. His mind had protectively blocked those years. Frank had learned dissociation as a method of survival. He said, "The only thing I remember was that I was happy the day my father died. The only grief I suffered was the fact that relatives were all over the house and I wanted to watch a TV show."

As Frank unraveled the memories of his traumatic childhood, he realized that some of the basis for his feelings continued to sabotage his adult relationships. He had lived in a tyrannical family in which rage and money were used to control. He still cannot recall much of his childhood, but a call to his mother confirmed his suspicions. His father had been a man full of rage. Most often, he took it out on Frank.

His mother related, "You made him even more enraged because you would not cry when he hit you. You just threw that little jaw out and looked at him defiantly. He thought you weren't listening to him or didn't care. So he hit you harder." Even in relating this story to Frank as an adult, his mother placed him in the position of being responsible for his father's rage, although, of course, in reality his father was an out-of-control adult.

Frank learned to retreat into his own quiet rage to protect himself emotionally from the abuse. His rage was a legitimate, healthy reaction to his father's beatings. His mind somehow decided he could heal from the blisters and bruises from the whippings. But he feared that if he expressed his feelings, his father might lose all control and kill him.

The emotional hurt of having someone who was supposed to love and protect him repeatedly abusing his body and soul was something too incredible for his young mind to comprehend. Frank's quiet rage served him well. It helped him survive emotionally, as a child. Holding onto his rage served as an emotional power source in an environment where his abusive father had all the control. His problems later in life came from his inability to associate the adult's eruptions of his core feelings to the hurt he felt as a child and then to work through how that abuse affected his viewpoints on life, his personal belief system, and his emotional development. Instead, Frank's disconnected feelings often came out sideways. He became unable to tell the difference between legitimate anger and rage triggered by core feelings, because he felt there was no safe expression or outlet for either. When the rage seemed ready to explode, he learned to eat.

As Frank got older, the intense rage did not go away. Instead, it became a stumbling block between him and any relationship he attempted. Constant rage left no room for other feelings. When love or trust began to surface, his old fears of abandonment would flood him until he felt inadequate. The branded messages of his childhood served as a barrier to the adult's happiness. Frank protected himself from getting too close to anyone. He spent sixty to seventy hours per week at his job, which met his programmed message that money equals power and also made him unavailable to anyone with healthy expectations. The women he chose for relationships were not emotionally available to him. Although he longed for closeness and acceptance in a loving relationship, he feared that he would once again be hurt if he allowed any vulnerability to sneak into his life. He became controlling and pushed away many healthy women. When a few persisted despite his sabotages, Frank felt driven to gain more weight. Although the added pounds did not push these women away, it provided a humiliating factor that isolated him in his loneliness. Ashamed to go out the door, ashamed to let a woman see his body, Frank reinforced his steel trap.

Frank is a gentle, caring man who for years shouldered an uncontrollable amount of rage—unaware of the reason. He never knew the whippings were extreme or that every boy had a right not to be hurt. In learning the origin of his feelings, he was able to stop their continued re-emergence as trauma bonds and to change the destructive messages he ultimately began to believe about himself. Today he does not have to summon a pizza in the middle of the night to block the feelings. He does not have to increase his weight to look or feel unattractive when he gets too close to a woman. He doesn't automatically reach for food anymore, although he admits that frequently food is his first want. Frank has found his way through the rage by identifying the reason for the hurt and anger underneath it and, then, confronting it with the same anger techniques you're learning. It was a journey a long time coming.

You may remember rage at the dinner table between your parents, or directed at you or your siblings. Exercising extreme control over your food as a child may have deflected adult tension. Because it was not safe for you to speak in your defense, food could become the mechanism to push down your own anger or to exert some control. You may have started to sneak food and eat as a means of rebellion. Or, if you were under constant scrutiny to eat everything, you may have learned to hide food in your napkin, under bread, or under potatoes to make your parents think you ate it all. Often people struggling with weight share stories of families who medicated their feelings with food after a huge and loud family argument.

But dangerous rages sometimes can be cold and silent. One woman recalled the fear she felt when tension began to increase in her home. The fear went off the scale when, one Sunday following church, her father parked the family car on railroad tracks in the path of an oncoming train and locked all the doors. He didn't say a word but sat coldly staring at her mother, who was too afraid to speak for fear her entire family would be lost. With only moments to spare and the train horn blaring a frantic warning, he started the car and drove home. The woman recalled, "Mom tried to make it all better by cooking a big Sunday feast. Not one word was said about the incident by anyone—ever, as far as I know. We just ate and ate, stuffing down our fear and hatred of this cold, cruel act. We all learned that we can expect to be hurt by people who say they love and care about you. We also learned that what we thought of as anger put our lives in jeopardy.

"I always thought that, if I let myself become angry, I would be just like my father," she continued. "The more I discounted my own anger, the more pounds I added.

"I thought I was afraid of anger, but what I really feared was his rage."

The Fear of Facing Your Fear

There is a strong foreboding associated with getting in touch with anger, which some picture as a black rage. There is fear that acknowledging anger will set off an out-of-control explosion. There is also a deeper fear if the people who hurt you are ones you love or want to be loved by; unrealistically, you may believe that if the pain is acknowledged, you will lose them and be alone. But remember, acknowledging that you had a justification for rage associated with an event provides you a key to accessing healthy anger and to releasing pain.

"If I acknowledged anger at my mother, I would be admitting that she hurt me," Becky confided. She feared showing her vulnerability, because as a child that usually just added to her pain. She preferred pushing down her hurt and anger. The consequences were a lifelong struggle with her weight and a low-grade depression that interfered with her ability to attain satisfaction in anything she attempted. She also feared that such an acknowledgment would force her into a face-to-face confrontation with her mother—something she was not ready for and did not necessarily have to do to become healthier.

Tools for Confronting Your Abuse

You can learn to confront your abuse by using a variety of techniques. Setting boundaries, being assertive, and acknowledging the truth are

tools you can safely use to make decisions about your family relationships. You alone will decide whether it would be beneficial to verbally
confront someone with your feelings regarding past abuse. It takes
emotional preparation for any confrontation. If you decide a person-
to-person confrontation is needed, your first step is to set clear, realistic goals that provide you with safeguards during and after such an
encounter. For example, if your goal is to get someone to apologize or
understand, you are setting yourself up for failure. A goal needs to be
something you know you can achieve, not something that is within
the other person's control. A realistic goal would be to break the
silence. Telling the truth would then be a successful confrontation.

You can add what you'll learn from the exercises later in this
chapter to the preparation you've already accomplished by attacking
trauma bonds, validating and expressing your feelings, and tossing out
negative messages. You've also learned to confront the interference of
past abuse in your daily life by practicing reality checks and by removing yourself from current abuse or manipulation.

Anger will continue to churn without some validation and interpretation of the confusing feelings. No matter what kind of happy
face you wear, anger will still control your life until you validate this
deep emotion, identify its causes, and take action. You may find you
can lose weight for a period of time. However, at some point you will
no longer be able to manage the anger you controlled with food. You
will tire of your attempts to white-knuckle the emotion. Instead, you
will turn your anger full force on the latest diet and sabotage your
efforts. Your latest attempt to eat more healthfully will take its place
among the graveyard of numerous unhealthful diets.

Examining Anger at Its Roots

Anger is a healthy emotion or feeling. It is our mind's way of telling us
to be careful, to protect ourselves. If you grew up in a family where rage
was a primary means of communication, it blurred the meaning of
anger and buried anger's true purpose by permeating your home with

fear. Therefore, it is crucial that you learn the difference between rage and anger and that you learn how both have affected you.

Examining anger at its roots is an important aspect of recovery. First, it is important to understand why anger has become such a very bad word. To illustrate this point, consider Becky's account: "Anger seemed so ugly," Becky said. "I was just not comfortable even thinking about it." Becky grew up in a home where her parents fought constantly. Occasionally, she witnessed her father become enraged and physically abusive toward her older brother. Within her environment, Becky learned it was not safe to express anger, and on the few times she attempted, the adults in her life made her believe that, instead of her anger being justified, she was the cause of any problem; if someone hurt her, it was because she deserved it, she was responsible. Her parents flooded her with negative messages. She was told she had no right to anger because she was the little girl who was bad, was never good enough, constantly proven wrong. With no one to validate the deep, churning emotion of anger, Becky discounted her pain. She attempted to repress her feelings as she cycled through various behaviors involving eating disorders. As a teenager, she purged the flood of anger with violence against herself in the form of vomiting, using laxatives, and bingeing. At other times, she restricted or controlled the amount of food she ate as she continued progressing toward what she secretly considered a slow, painfully deserved death. As an adult, she began to overeat.

Trained to emotionally restrain her anger in the form of guilt, Becky spent much of her life absorbing the pain of others and trying to make things right. She learned to make a joke when people said hurtful things about her appearance. Crippling sarcasm wounded her to the core. Yet, she made fun of herself and became an accomplice to the pain. Tears were pushed down with overeating, not eating, or purging. Anger was resisted or redirected with this movement.

Becky learned to say her apologies quickly because the emotion she allowed herself to feel the most was guilt, although it was frequently undeserved. Even if she believed momentarily that she had a right to be angry, ultimately she was persuaded that her actions in some way provoked the pain inflicted by others. "I never believed I was entitled to be angry. I was taught that everything that has happened to me has been my fault. I can't blame anyone for that."

How Anger Has Been Expressed in Your Life

Healthy families acknowledge anger and seek peaceful resolutions. We all say things we do not mean from time to time. However, in healthy families, that person can make amends by apologizing and by not repeating the offensive behavior again. That's important to remember, because some people never change their behavior and habitually try to avoid responsibility by saying "I'm sorry." Healthy families focus on addressing behaviors that make them angry, not on making the person who expresses anger feel bad or unworthy.

Examining the influences of your environment on your expressions of anger and rage provides you with several levels of understanding. First, you'll gain more empathy and, hopefully, respect for how you coped as a child in a difficult environment. You'll continue to reduce the self-blame and negative core messages that have consistently pulled you down when you have attempted to eat healthfully. Second, you'll recognize that you do not have to make the same mistakes as others and that, even if you have, you can change by combining the new techniques you're learning in this chapter with others you've learned about owning and expressing feelings. Third, in facing your fear of anger, you have seen that the worst is over. You can move through it because knowledge is always power.

Completing the Family Expressions of Anger exercise which follows will help you further identify why you have been afraid of anger. The next time you get angry, you'll be able to use everything you have learned in your steps thus far. You'll know how not to back down but how to examine why you are angry before you make a decision regarding what action to take next. If you're overreacting to a core feeling and distorted perceptions, you have learned how to confront these and not reach for food to push the anger away.

Use this exercise to further investigate how your family patterns have influenced your holding back anger. Also, take an honest look to see if you exhibit some of these same patterns. If you do, consider these as red flags because they often will be connected to destructive eating.

Underneath each family member, identify how that person exhibited anger. For example, did your mother threaten to leave the house, was she assertive, or did she scream? Did your father drink when he was angry, or did he sit down and talk to the person he was angry with? Consider the example below, before you begin completing your unique family experience chart.

Family Expressions of Anger Exercise			
Example: My Family of Childhood Unhealthy Expressions of Anger			
Father	**Mother**	**Sibling**	**Grandparent**
Yells	Beatings	Isolates	Withholds affection
Blames	Martyr	Martyr	Blames Cold silence
Evil looks	Manipulates	Drinks	Manipulates Looks Controls
Threats	Withdraws	Runs away	Threatens to leave
Controls	Eats	Controls	Restricts food
Example: My Family of Childhood Healthy Expressions of Anger			
Father	**Mother**	**Sibling**	**Grandparent**

Talks to me
    about what makes
    him angry with me
	Assertiveness
	Discusses what
	    happened
		Talks to me
		    directly
		Doesn't call
			Assertive
			Doesn't hold
			    grudges

Listens to what I
    have to say
	Problem-solves
	Focuses on behavior
		me names	Tries to decrease
			    his anger by

Does not make me
    feel I am a bad person
	Talks directly to the
	    person she is angry with
			facing it, doesn't
			    escalate it

Family Expressions of Anger Exercise			
Example: My Family of Childhood Expressions of Anger			
Father	**Mother**	**Sibling**	**Grandparent**
Example: My Family Expressions of Anger Today			
Father	**Mother**	**Sibling**	**Grandparent**

Continue your exploration by charting how those close to you as an adult express their anger or rage. Do you see any similarities with your family of origin?

Adult Patterns of Anger Expression				
Boyfriends	**Girlfriends**	**Spouse**	**Bosses**	**Children**

1. After completing the exercises, circle behaviors that were experienced in rage, not anger.
2. Identify the behaviors of rage or anger that triggered your eating or restricting food when you were a child.
3. Identify the behaviors of rage or anger that trigger your eating or restricting food today.

You cannot complete this process honestly without accessing how you yourself express anger, a process that you'll do in the following exercise. In completing it, you may discover unhealthy similarities that make you uncomfortable. Instead of falling into self-blame, take heart. You have decided to make changes in your life, and your work thus far indicates you are doing just that. Now you know how unhealthy reactions can affect people you care about, and you've also learned alternative ways to communicate.

My Expressions of Anger			
As a Child	**As a Teenager**	**As an Adult**	**As an Adult in Recovery**

This exercise can be quite an eye-opener. You may discover you have married someone who has traits just like the person you feared the most when growing up. Or, you may discover your own similar traits. Finally, after completing the exercise, it is probably easier for you to see why you may have started to use food to try to control anger.

What Are Your Roadblocks to Expressing Anger?

As you have discovered, it is crucial to identify roadblocks that keep you from making the progress you want. As we discussed, fear of family reactions to your changes can stop you cold unless you face your fear head on. Use the following statements and questions to help you address what is holding you back and to stimulate you to consider ways to move aside the stumbling blocks.

Identifying Barriers

1. I'm afraid to acknowledge my anger because

2. What is the worst possible thing that could happen if I acknowledge my anger?
3. What is the best possible thing that could happen?
4. What messages would I expect or fear from my family if I began to validate my anger?
    a.
    b.
    c.
5. Would I accept those as reasons not to validate anger if they were said by anyone else? (If yes, please specify why beside each response.)
6. What programmed core messages do I give myself to prevent a healthy expression of anger?
    a.
    b.
    c.
7. What replacement messages can I give myself that will allow me to acknowledge and express my anger?

As you completed the questions, you used a process that is helpful in problem solving and facing any fear. By following this progression of questions, you'll often bring forward answers you held inside but were not confident enough to act upon. This process demonstrates that you have hidden capabilities and that you will benefit if you routinely stop, face your fears, investigate them and listen to yourself.

Taking Action When You're Angry

Now that you know it's okay to be angry, what do you do with it? It is probably very easy for you to be angry with yourself. It may even be easy for you to become angry with the garbage collector or the person who cuts in front of you in traffic. However, you may need some help allowing yourself to become angry at the destructive behaviors of people who are most important, people you care about or even love. When you are angry with them, you want to take action to protect yourself, either by voluntarily leaving a volatile situation or by assertively confronting it.

It's not as easy as it sounds. You, like many others, may think it is most important and even easier to forgive someone and then to try to forget your hurt and anger. However, if you do that first, most likely those feelings will continue to interfere not only as unclaimed emotions inside of you but as emotions that stand between you and a closer relationship with that person. For example, you may say you forgive someone, but it will be extremely difficult to trust that person again unless you claim the hurt and take action to protect yourself from it happening to you again. If you use the anger techniques that follow, you have an opportunity to clarify any distortions and solve problems. You'll find that, by releasing the anger, you'll be much more able to forgive and have a closer relationship.

On the other hand, anger and resentment can bind you closely to someone you choose never to be a part of your life due to physical or emotional safety. When you are able to own the anger, and then let it go, you can find peace.

Anger Techniques That Make a Difference

Choose one of the following techniques to help you practice the healthy expression of anger. The first will help you challenge core messages that may hinder your taking care of yourself. The second technique is assertiveness, a skill you will find yourself using daily. The third and fourth techniques, writing a confrontation letter and the Anger Workout Steps, focus on taking the power away from past behaviors that still hurt and anger you.

Changing Core Messages

Using what you know about core messages, think about any messages that might stop you from freely releasing your hurt and anger. You'll need to tackle these first, or you will find your experience in the following exercises to be stilted and incomplete. Review the destructive core messages and potential replacement messages in the following example.

Example	
Old Destructive Core Message	*Powerful Replacement*
1. You should not be angry.	1. I have a right to my anger.
2. Your hurt is not real.	2. I am hurt. I can take care of me.
3. Do not talk.	3. I have a right to be heard.
4. You are betraying the family.	4. I have been betrayed and I will not continue to accept it by feeling disloyal.
5. I can understand why he or she hurt me. I was bad. He was drinking.	5. There is no justifiable reason for anyone to hurt me.
6. If I show anger he or she will know I am vulnerable and hurt me more.	6. I am an adult now and can get away from people who hurt me.

Note your own destructive messages in the first column of your chart. You have learned a wealth of knowledge since you began with Step 1. Use talkback messages and affirmations you've learned about to write a powerful, positive replacement in the second column.

Changing Core Messages About Anger	
Old Destructive Core Message	*Powerful Replacement*

Now copy your old destructive message on one side of an index card and your powerful replacement message on the other side. Complete as many cards as necessary. Carry these with you in your wallet or briefcase. Review the cards when you have a break, but, most important, catch yourself the next time you hear that core message play in your head. Flip out the card and reinforce the replacement message by reading it aloud. Now that you have tackled the core feelings that have kept you silent when you've been angry, you're ready to practice assertiveness, a tool that really can empower you.

Assertiveness: The Power Tool
It sounds simple, but becoming assertive takes practice. At first, it may seem stilted, and you may find yourself fumbling with words a bit. But don't worry; that's part of the learning curve. You don't have to be perfect. You'll find that by changing the ways you approach your communication, you'll not only be able to express your anger but you will become much more effective in voicing all your thoughts, feelings, and needs.

One of the easiest techniques to use when practicing assertiveness is to complete the following three sentences:
  1. I think . . .
  2. I feel . . .
  3. I need . . .

Now, here's the hard part. In the first and second sentence, you cannot use the word YOU. If you do, the person you are talking to will automatically become defensive and is less likely to listen to what you have to say. The purpose of your first sentence is to clarify what the problem is. That's helpful to you and the other person. You can't solve a problem unless you know what it is.

In the second sentence, express three feelings. If you express only one feeling, that may not describe the total picture of what is going on. For instance, if you express the feelings of anger, hurt, and frustration, the person you are talking to may be more inclined to listen because you have shared some vulnerability in saying you are hurt, and most people can relate to that. And if one of those feelings is a core feeling, it is a message to yourself to proceed with caution. Step back and make sure you are not reacting to a trauma bond. You'll also find it hard just to state the three feelings, and not include the word "that." If you say "I feel that," you are making a thinking statement, and it is almost impossible not to add the accusing word "you" afterwards. You might as well be pointing your finger in someone's face. Think about how you would feel. The purpose of the second step is also to heighten your knowledge of your own feelings and to increase the empathy of the other person toward you.

In the third step, you clearly state what you need. As you go through this process in order, you may also realize what you want is different from what you need. If absolutely necessary, you can cheat a little and use the word "you" in the third sentence.

When you are beginning, follow the format exactly. Be sure to limit yourself to the three sentences. Keep it simple. If you begin to add sentences and feel a need to talk in paragraphs, you'll find you are either lecturing or defending yourself and have moved away from the assertiveness technique. Regroup and begin again.

If you use these assertiveness tools on a regular basis, you'll find that you will be taking care of yourself routinely and that you will have fewer reasons to be angry. You certainly won't fall back into the habit of repressing your anger. You won't have to raise your voice to use this effective tool to express anger, and you won't have to worry about hurting someone else's feelings, because you are taking ownership of your thoughts and feelings with "I" statements and not making hurtful accusations. You are simply stating the need to solve a problem. The following examples will give you an idea how to clearly state the problem, express your feelings, and describe what you need.

Assertiveness Example

Joely dreaded going out to dinner with her husband, because he always seemed to focus on what she ate. Although he did this focusing under the auspices of caring about her, she felt hurt. Ignoring that hurt and staying silent were forms of self-betrayal that made her revert into her old core feeling of not being good enough. In order to confront those feelings and not revert to her old coping mechanism of overeating, she had to stand up for herself assertively. Here's how she spoke to her husband about her concern.

"I think I can make choices about what I eat."

"I feel frustrated, hurt, and angry."

"I need you to stop pointing out how many calories are in the foods I eat."

Joely also found it difficult to set boundaries and to say no to people, even if it made her overextend herself and neglect her own needs. Before she started using assertiveness techniques, Joely would stall, for fear she would hurt the person or because undeserved guilt led her to believe it was something she should do. This stalling set her up for continuous queries, because she did not definitively say no. After practicing at home what she would say at an upcoming meeting at church, Joely was able to use her new skills in setting boundaries when a woman in the meeting would not take no for an answer to her request for Joely to teach Bible School.

"I think I have said that this year I do not have time."

"I'm feeling frustrated, angry, and pressured."

"I need not to be asked again."

Using assertiveness techniques doesn't always mean that the other person will respond as you would want. However, each time you are assertive, you take control and assume responsibility. You increase the potential for change substantially and reduce the tendency to expect someone else to read your mind in order to respond to your needs. You'll come away from a conversation feeling confident that you have not run away from a problem, or left behind misunderstandings and hurt that can build to increasing anger. Practicing assertiveness daily will increase your self-confidence overall, and practicing assertiveness is an effective way to continuously practice integrating the needs of your head and your heart.

Releasing Anger Through Writing

Writing can be another powerful release of thoughts and feelings. You can keep a daily journal, or you can write a letter to a person with whom you are angry. Don't worry about how that person or others will react, because it is a confrontation letter that does not need to be mailed. While you write the letter, don't be concerned about anything other than expressing your raw thoughts and emotions. The letter's purpose is to acknowledge and release your own hurt. As you may recall from chapter 7, on loss, we discussed how it is sometimes easier to assume the blame for someone else's actions than to place responsibility where it belongs. Acknowledging your pain takes courage and does not make you a victim; if you ignore its consequences, you continue to be a victim of the past.

Today, identify one person's behavior and stay focused on that person until you complete the letter and any subsequent revisions. Remember, this is a process of safely releasing anger, not rage. Let yourself stop the exercise at any time, thus setting your boundaries. However, if you stop, be sure to analyze why you are having difficulties, and then set a time frame for going back to complete it.

In the past, ambiguities and vagueness may have kept you anxious and unsettled and may have interfered with your ability to stay on task. However, as you've progressed through the steps related to core feelings, messages, and anger, you have successfully been able to focus and have not allowed yourself to be sidetracked. Those sidetracks can take you away from facing the real problem and can make all problems much bigger than they are. Because letting go of repressed anger is crucial to ending your weight problems, it is important that you follow through with all aspects of the next two exercises.

The purpose of these last two exercises, writing a confrontation letter and completing the Anger Workout Steps, is not to figure out why someone hurt you but to wrench out and let go of deeply buried core feelings. In this process, you will gain empathy for yourself and, hopefully, some self-forgiveness. As we discussed earlier, forgiveness of yourself and others is more lasting if it is given after you honestly honor your own feelings.

While these examples may not seem applicable to you, everyone gets angry. You can benefit from completing these exercises, whether it helps you connect to and release repressed anger, or increases your confidence in maintaining control when you express anger, a healthy emotion.

Here is the process:

1. Write exactly how you feel. It is only for you. No one will sit in judgment of how grammatically correct it is. Your feelings are essential. Let them rip. Most people start this exercise by scheduling 10 to 30 minutes to write a general letter, pouring out their feelings. Do not be slowed by a concentration on neatness or whether it makes sense. There is no right or wrong, no perfect letter to complete.

2. Don't spend time now attempting to figure out why someone hurt you with his or her behavior. It would not take long for that person's voice to interject into your writing. Instead of an anger letter to someone who harmed you, it becomes an instrument of self-shame and repulsion. Consequently, reframe statements such as "How could you?" and "Why did you?" There really is no legitimate reason to hurt someone, especially a child or an adult in a vulnerable situation

3. Don't make excuses for the person to whom you are directing anger. It is time to stop accepting that it is okay for someone

to hurt you, as long as there is a reasonable explanation. You would not accept that excuse for yourself. In this letter, your job is to express thoughts and feelings you have repressed. Be specific with instances that made you angry. Remember, voicing healthy anger does not mean you are abandoning a relationship.

4. Allow yourself to be entitled to your anger. Make clear statements and follow them with a "because," such as "I am angry with you for telling me it was my fault you were unhappy because I grew up being attracted to other depressed people I thought I should fix ... I am angry with you for stealing my childhood because you kept me away from other children for fear I would tell our family secrets. I am angry with you for touching me and making me feel dirty but telling me you loved me at the same time, because I have grown up thinking it is okay for people who love me to hurt me ... I am angry at you for leaving me with Mom because you knew she was drunk and might hurt me again. . . . I am angry because you never spent any time with me unless you were abusing me. . . . I am angry with you because you tried to make me into an adult when I was only a child. . . . I am angry with you because you always focused on my weight. . . . I am angry with you because you always found something wrong with my grades. . . . I am angry with you because I always had to be perfect. . . . I am angry with you because you ignored me."

   Or, if you are expressing anger at an experience, you might state something like "I am angry at being hyperactive, because I was always labeled a troublemaker and didn't fit in."

Let this list go on as long as you can. It is safe. There is no one to stop you unless you choose to let someone else (alive or dead) dictate your movements. Consider this a work in progress. Choose to set healthy boundaries for yourself. If you become overwhelmed at any time, take breaks to ground yourself, use reality checks, affirmations, and other techniques you have already learned.

This exercise also can be very empowering. Take time to pat yourself on the back for finally expressing deep feelings. Anger can be very healing and empowering. You are releasing it slowly, as if releasing the valve on a pressure cooker. If you are in therapy, share this letter with your therapist.

After you write your first letter, read it aloud. Then read it again with feeling. The more anger you can express verbally, the more it will feel comfortable to you and not an overwhelming burden turned into guilt. Always be specific. Don't get lost in a storm cloud of pain. Rewrite it, being even more specific. It may take several times before you can cleanse yourself of the anger.

One letter will not release all your pain or anger. Continue letting go by using this process again whenever you need it in your life.

Working Anger Out

The Anger Workout Steps that follows walk you through a five-step process to identify behaviors that have hurt you, to increase your self-empathy and ability to care for yourself, and to help you arrive at an affirmation statement that replaces old core feelings. Notice that the process allows you to step back and look at the facts around a situation. While you may have been the victim of an abusive situation, the Anger Workout Steps will empower you to let go of any long-lasting residue.

Completing the steps also helps you establish a more natural reaction and progression to help you acknowledge and let go of anger immediately when something hurts you. It teaches you an unfiltered process that allows you to react strongly to a hurt and then move through it. What you'll experience in this exercise is the same process many people go through mentally, yet may not complete to its entirety with an affirmation.

By progressing through each step in order, you are able to let go of anger quickly and completely. First, you are acknowledging the behavior that hurt you; second, you are immediately expressing your feelings; third, you're stepping back with a reality assessment that prevents you from assuming responsibility for your own hurt or simply ignoring it to avoid acknowledging that a particular person would hurt you; fourth, you are giving yourself a primal voice with your power statement; and finally, you conclude by further taking care of your needs with a soothing affirmation that directly addresses your hurt.

Compare that to your old ways of processing anger that probably would have concluded with your using food. Make extra copies of the Anger Workout Steps, because you'll find the process helpful in the final stages of letting go of trauma bonds and loss, too. You'll be surprised at the feelings of empowerment, release and calmness you'll feel after you complete the Anger Workout Steps for each traumatic event and loss.

Exercise: Anger Workout Steps

Note: You may find it helpful to substitute *hurt* for *anger* initially because hurt is underneath all anger.

I. Identify the behavior or experience that made you angry:

I felt angry (hurt) when you . . .

2. How did it make you feel?

It made me feel . . .

Continue with your feelings beneath the anger such as hurt, confusion, worthlessness. (How many are core feelings that trigger eating today?)

3. Reality Check: I was only ___ years old. A ___ year-old child should not be expected to . . .

This is your reality statement. It helps to examine what happened by looking at expectations. For example, would a five-year-old child be capable developmentally of performing the task you were punished for not getting done perfectly? Is that a healthy expectation from a parent or sibling? Write a statement describing how someone should have acted. For example, "A child should be able to expect protection from her father.... Parents should make a child feel secure.... Adults should not sexually use children.... A child should not expect his relationship with his parents to always be based on performance.... A child should be able to go out and play and not be stuck in a hospital.... A child shouldn't be labeled as bad because the chemicals in his body cause him to have attention deficit disorder and make it difficult for him to be still."

4. Power Statement: You had no right! . . .
Talk back in this statement. Follow your statements in this section with an exclamation point. Say anything you feel from your heart. Say those things you have been afraid to say or thought were inappropriate. No one judges this statement. Work to get rid of your anger.

5. Affirmation: I deserve (to be heard, protected, wanted, etc . . .).
This statement should be very specific to the incident of anger you are writing about. Make this a working affirmation you will use daily to replace the old shame feelings. If you have followed the Anger Workout Steps in progression, a unique affirmation that meets your needs will probably flow out naturally at their conclusion. For example, if you were told to be quiet every time you spoke or if you were slapped when you disagreed with your parent, you were programmed to believe you were not entitled to speak. Your affirmation might be "I deserve to be heard. What I say is important. I am important."

The Food Connection
If you examine your anger in terms of your use of food and your weight concerns, you will discover that the feelings beneath the anger are the same ones connected with your emotionally driven eating, bingeing, purging, or restricting food episodes. Often these are feelings that make you believe you are bad.

Use the same anger techniques you learned in this chapter with a few minor changes, substituting your weight or body image as an object of your anger for another person's behavior. It is a helpful way to reduce your own denial concerning your anger's impact. Completing this exercise with weight as the focus can actually reduce your need to use food as a means to repress anger or rebellion or as a way to get power. Although several reasons for anger are shown below, when you do the exercise, focus on only one reason at a time. Otherwise it will be too easy for you to become distracted from what is your real source of anger and thus, the exercise will not be effective. It also is likely that each one will lead you to different reality checks, affirmations, and power statements.

For example:

1. What Makes Me Angry?

   I feel angry I can't find an attractive bathing suit. I feel angry because I gain weight so easily, and other people seem to eat whatever they want.

2. How Does it Make Me Feel? It makes me feel like I'm an oddball, like I don't fit in anywhere when I go swimming. I feel paranoid, as if everyone is looking at me. I feel unaccepted, rejected, and automatically judged because of my weight. I feel cheated and irritated because I gain weight more easily than others.
   Reality Check:

   I should be able to buy a bathing suit that is colorful and trendy. Just because I am not as skinny as a model doesn't mean I should be punished for it and not have the selection others do. And I have a right to be irritated because other people don't work as hard as I do, yet seem to have no weight problems. The reality is, it isn't fair that some people can have more freedom in what they eat and that it doesn't show up in pounds. It is not that I am a lazy person. It just means we are made differently or different things in my life have affected my use of food. While I am working to change the things I can, I may have genes and hormones that influence my weight, as well. I have to focus on what I can and want to change. I can't change that fact that other people have fewer problems with their weight. I can acknowledge that it stinks!

3. Power statement:

It's wrong for me to be discriminated against or judged because of my weight! Being overweight is not a moral issue! There are lots of different things involved. No one has a right to judge me without getting to know me first!

4. Affirmation:

I deserve the same rights and considerations as a thin person. My weight does not change who I am inside.

Keep working. Keep letting go. If you still feel intense anger after completing the anger exercises and can think of no more reasons to be angry, you may want to continue with some experiential methods to release the anger from your body. Running, hitting a punching bag or pillow, and screaming in the shower are only a few. These are ineffective alone. Therefore, always connect to the reason for the anger by using these methods after you have completed your written exercises. If your anger persists, dig deeper, using what you have learned about trauma bonds and loss. Keep working until you identify your anger's origin and let it go.

Your anger is valid. It has been built up and directed inward or misdirected as a loose cannon for some time. You are making a significant step in your recovery by directing the anger toward a behavior or its point of origin.

Releasing repressed anger can sometimes make you physically sick. If you become sick, acknowledge that it is probably your body's reaction to letting go of capped pain. Tell yourself that this pain would have remained trapped inside, propelling you to hurt yourself, if you had not taken action. Nurture yourself through any sickness. Meet your needs. If you need a physician, contact one. You will find that demonstrating you can take care of your needs is very healing.

Anger also can provide a warm, peaceful release. Capture that feeling and remember it.

Building a Safety Net

Above all, make sure you are safe. Never drive a car when you are angry. Build safe boundaries to ensure that children do not become the brunt of your anger. Feelings of pain you have held for years can go away when you learn to use the safe tools of recovery. Plan your writing during a quiet time, alone. Build a safe boundary for your work. Limit the time to no more than thirty minutes at a sitting. If you fall into old patterns and again direct the anger inward, stop the process until you can seek professional help. Your therapist may allow you to complete anger exercises at his or her office. If you ever think about hurting yourself during your recovery process or become suicidal, seek the help of a professional immediately. Your life is one to be valued.

Awareness Sparks Change

In recognizing the reasons and depths of your own anger, you probably have improved your insight into the actions of others. You may have become aware of times when you became enraged and lost control, hurting others. Make amends and let it go. Always remember anger is meant to be a momentary emotion that directs us to take care of ourselves, either by choosing to leave a dangerous situation or by being assertive. Your progression through these anger exercises has demonstrated that you have the guts to look deep inside and take ownership of some feelings and thoughts that you may have discounted and hidden.

Now that you have tackled the difficult emotional connections to eating, you're ready to explore how chemical reactions within your body can also influence your appetite and weight.

AFFIRMATION

Today I'll tune into the reasons for my anger,
focus on positive ways to let myself be heard,
and let the anger go.

9

RECOGNIZING THE CHEMICAL FACTOR

Always be encouraged. It's often the last key
on the bunch that unlocks the door.

—Anonymous

The food industry spends thousands of dollars each year to find out what triggers the need to eat compulsively, and it is paying more and more attention to the chemistry of the brain. The link between internal body chemistry and insatiable cravings for food, alcohol, and cocaine is one of the reasons that typical diets don't have long-term success.

Mental health professionals know that chemical changes in the body can affect emotional health, too. Recently, much has been said about a possible change in the body chemistry of those who are under chronic stress or who have undergone traumatic experiences—two common elements in the lives of people with food and weight problems. While there is much to learn about the link between chemical reactions and food, you may be able to use what has already been discovered.

Step 8: Recognize the presence of chemical reactions that affect your weight.

Chemicals produced in the brain can affect appetite and cravings. For example, some people with weight issues state emphatically that they do not binge on a particular food. But when they analyze their eating patterns, they are surprised to discover that eating that particular food is the trigger that precipitates a binge or purge. In other words, a specific food caused a chemical reaction that led to the binge or purge.

For instance, one woman said she never ate more than a cup or two of potato chips. Yet within a few hours of eating the chips she would begin to crave chocolate. She believed that eating the first bite of chocolate precipitated the subsequent binge and did not connect the chips with her binge. However, when she examined her pattern, she began to believe that eating chips instigated a chemical reaction that triggered chocolate cravings and propelled her into a binge. It was a cycle leading to shame, guilt, depression, hopelessness, and low self-esteem. And, of course, she said she felt disgustingly fat. Identifying the connection, however, allowed her to break that cycle.

The Brain's Chemical Messengers: Neurotransmitters

Neurotransmitters are chemical substances that transmit nerve impulses within the brain; each neurotransmitter is designed to fit into a particular receptor on the surface of a brain cell, conveying information that either prompts or inhibits continued impulses or actions in the body. In the human brain, there are about 100 neurotransmitters that perform a variety of functions. Research has indicated neurotransmitters regulate appetite for fats, proteins, and carbohydrates. They are also linked to feelings. Some people may have an abnormally low level of certain neurotransmitters, thereby inhibiting or slowing important messages, or an overproduction that results in depression, appetite suppression, and cravings. Let's look at three neurotransmitters, as well as some amino acids (which are neurotransmitter precursors) that have been linked to appetite.

Dopamine

Have you ever eaten as a reward? Some neurotransmitters such as dopamine are associated with the feelings generated when you reward yourself.

Dopamine also inhibits hunger, as scientists studying cocaine have found. Through their research, they have discovered much about dopamine's role in appetite suppression, since one of cocaine's side effects is the inhibition of appetite. Cocaine binds to proteins that normally transport dopamine and prevents their re-uptake, or normal progression. Dopamine levels increase, and dopamine remains active longer, continually stimulating neurons and causing prolonged feelings of pleasure. Researchers theorize eating certain foods causes this same reaction.

Serotonin

Serotonin is the body's calming neurotransmitter, regulating a sense of well-being and motivation. When you ingest carbohydrates, serotonin levels increase, giving you a positive change of mood. The rise in serotonin is caused by the body's increased level of tryptophan, an amino acid.

If your body does not have enough serotonin, you may load up on carbohydrates as an unhealthy way to self-treat depression or anxiety. One theory for why carbohydrates bring a feeling of well-being is that when you eat a starch, the body converts it to sugar, and sugar then stimulates the pancreas to release insulin. Insulin triggers a rise in tryptophan. A more healthful way to increase the body's level of tryptophan is to eat foods that of themselves are high in it: bananas, chicken, tofu, turkey, and pineapple, among others. Combining these tryptophan-rich foods with carbohydrates enables your brain to absorb tryptophan more effectively; you benefit from having a higher level of serotonin without the extra pounds from too many carbohydrates.

Research also has suggested that serotonin is the brain chemical that stimulates feelings of power. In studies, animals given a drug that boosted serotonin levels showed an extreme rise in confidence. Other studies show that dominant males in animal societies tend to have high levels of serotonin. Some researchers, drawing the parallel between animals and humans, believe that people in positions of corporate power may actually have higher serotonin levels than the rest of us. If you lower their serotonin level, they lose that edge. It makes sense then, that people with a history of dysfunctional use of food will reach for foods high in carbohydrates when struggling to get some control in their lives. Food gives a momentary sense of control or power. Sales of prescription drugs designed to stimulate serotonin activity have surged. Although a pill may reduce appetite and stimulate a temporary feeling of well-being, it still will not take away the emotional origins that will perpetuate the cycle.

Endorphins

Do you know people who eat sweets when they are depressed? They may be unconsciously reaching for the mood-altering effect of endorphins, which function as nature's morphine. These neurotransmitters are chemically similar to opium. Endorphins contribute to the calm feeling some people experience after bingeing or purging and to the euphoria of a runner's high.

Scientists tell us that endorphin levels increase for those under stress and that these endorphins actually boost the craving for fat and protein. Under normal circumstances, fats and protein help the body restore energy. But in a binge combined with chronic stress (a normal situation for those with long-term food and weight issues), the body does not get an opportunity to balance out. Some evidence suggests that severe food restriction increases endorphins; therefore, an anorexic starting to increase eating could suffer like a heroin addict in withdrawal. That effect possibly explains the difficulty in intervening successfully with someone in a compulsive overexercising mode.

Amino Acids

Studies have shown that the use of amino acid precursors of neurotransmitters, like tryptophan, can be beneficial in reducing cravings.

The presence of amino acids is necessary to activate glands and to act as chemical switches that control metabolism and other body functions. Some amino acids are generated within the body; others are made available through food. Amino acid supplements, which are also beneficial to those who suffer from low blood sugar, may be purchased in health food stores.

Before taking any amino acid supplement, consult with your doctor or nutritionist for individualized recommendations and ascertain a healthy dosage for your body. Taking too much can be dangerous. Tryptophan as a supplement was withdrawn by the U.S. Food and Drug Administration (FDA) in 1989 when several hundred people developed flu-like symptoms after taking it. Although it was widely thought people became ill from a contaminated batch, it remains unavailable in supplement form due to potentially adverse reactions.

Phenylalanine is another amino acid. It governs the release of cholecystokinin (CCK), an intestinal hormone that signals the brain to feel full and satisfied after eating. Your nutritionist may be able to direct you to other supplements that will be helpful.

Other Factors in Weight Loss

Still more research is being conducted on the "rush" some people feel from living on the edge. Why is one person energized by a crisis or the risk of death while another is terrorized? How does living in such an environment during childhood affect long-term chemical changes in the body? We know that one way the body reacts to stress is by secreting the hormone cortisol. Research indicates that this hormone can actually increase appetite. Often, the weight from that increase is distributed in the abdomen. Meditation to reduce stress may actually help you lose weight if you are on cortisol overload.

There has been some indication that you can alter chemical imbalances in your body by combining care of your body and spirit, which you have been doing. You are in a stage of recovery when you know that the binge or purge just doesn't work for you anymore.

Could that be because your work in recovery has actually altered the chemical imbalance and helped you reclaim your body? Much research is needed in this area, but it certainly holds promise for those suffering from chronic food issues related to trauma.

The research on the chemicals within the human body is starting to validate what those who have struggled with their weight have known for a long time: weight control is a much more complex task than steadfastly maintaining a new diet. It involves much more than willpower.

Now that your work has resulted in your ability today to connect your life events, feelings, and thoughts with your body's chemical reactions, you're ready to proceed to the next step: defining your own food strategy. In chapter 10, you're going to learn more about physical influences that affect what you eat, and why you have reactions to certain foods. With that information, you will want to throw away all your old diet plans and take complete control of your food choices.

AFFIrmaTIon
Today, as I untie my life's gifts,
I understand the intricate workings of my body.

| **10** |

STRATEGIC EATING

He who knows others is wise;
He who knows himself is enlightened.

—Lao-tzu

Does the thought of starting another diet plunge you into your Cycle of Pain? Hope. Lost pounds. Frustration. Scales of betrayal. Feeling that you are a failure. The belief that anyone who has enough stamina and willpower can lose pounds and keep them off simply by adhering to the newest diet is a surefire way to keep the Cycle of Pain in control of your life.

A few years ago, folks in the eating disorder treatment field decided they would direct people away from this cycle by calling diets "food plans." Although food plans provided the structure many desired, they still provoked the feel of a diet. Sometimes the sense of failure was even worse. People complained of feeling that they had no control in their lives when the food plan was dictated as a necessity. The feelings of no control and failure are two strong triggers to the Cycle of Pain.

One of the most dangerous feelings that diets can spark within you is that of deprivation. When that feeling begins to envelop you, it's usually not long before you reach for the forbidden. It is natural. When diets are too rigid and deprive us of what we want, our minds focus on what we cannot have. As the focus becomes more obsessive, the cravings tend to escalate. Reaching for that food can initially bring you a sense of power and a feeling that you have regained control.

A strict food plan can catapult you into a sense of shame and guilt because you're unable to adhere to it every moment. Then when you "slip" and taste that food that is not allowed, it can push you into a "what the heck" mode, prompting more eating and a sense of hopelessness or failure. As you have learned, unless you intervene with grounding techniques, reality checks, talkback, and other tools you have been practicing, the Cycle of Pain wins again.

However, you have started to alter the game plan. Tying emotions to food and learning how to change old patterns are powerful interventions. Reframing how you look at healthful eating and eliminating the power struggle between yourself and the next miracle diet are more strategic moves that you have integrated into your life now. Your work has prepared you for this important step of letting go of old standby diets and designing your own plan of eating. Like most people with weight issues, you probably know more than the average person about nutrition. And now that you've progressed through eight of the ten steps in the book, you have even more powerful knowledge of how your unique emotions and thoughts play into your use of food.

Step 9: Choose a strategic plan of eating that meets your needs and lifestyle.
Whether you simply approach eating in a more relaxed manner or design your own version of a structured plan, it is extremely important that you take the driver's seat now and stop turning over the wheel to others who promise they know what is best for you.

Get Rid of the Last Roadblocks
If you still have difficulty in making a choice that's right for you, don't despair. You may need to go back and dig a little deeper to discover what is keeping you stuck by really examining what purpose the excess pounds may be serving today. Weight also can serve as a protective layer. You can feel "safe at being left alone" if you feel fat or if you "disappear" by not eating. If you have been sexually abused,

you may be trying to use your weight as a signal to ward off any physical attraction. That's why many are stuck at a "safe" weight and never go lower. They self-sabotage when their weight decreases and feel vulnerable because others are now noticing their bodies. Invisibility is no longer an option. They have lost the illusion of safety from sexual advances that the weight provided. If you are anorexic, you may have continued to lose weight in an effort to disappear and protect yourself.

One woman whose weight had been stable for several months discovered that she was not losing more pounds because she did not want her mother, who had focused on her weight since she was a child, to think she had "won." She believed losing more pounds would put her at a disadvantage in that relationship. Once she had that understanding, she was able to examine more closely what was preventing her relationship with her mother from improving, without relying on her weight as a safety net. She reviewed her knowledge of trauma bonds and owning her feelings before she realized that she was stuck because she was still afraid of the unexpressed anger toward her mother. Using that information, she reworked the anger exercises in chapter 8 and slowly began setting her boundaries and expressing her anger with her mother. Then she was able to lose the lingering pounds.

As you've examined your life and relationships, you've also done a lot of work to increase your understanding and to put aside the roadblocks to losing weight and accepting yourself as a whole person, regardless of the scales. If you're stuck, it simply means you're ready to move on to your next level of understanding and tackle a problem that would have been too difficult before you had a solid experience of using the tools you have learned.

Eating Strategies: It's Your Choice

This chapter includes several eating strategies for you to choose from. There is no magic strategy for everyone. Review these and take bits and pieces to accommodate your unique emotional and physical needs. You may want to meet with a nutritionist for professional assistance and for fine-tuning your plan.

As long as you look at these strategies as your choice, there is no trigger to the Cycle of Pain. You may find the best strategy is one of bargaining. Become conscious of what you eat, and then increase or decrease your intake of fat, sugar, carbohydrates, and so on based on your overall daily food choices. This balance eliminates the sense of being deprived or of being different from others. It puts you squarely in the driver's seat—an extremely important position because many with weight problems had choices taken away from them.

For example, if you are going to a favorite restaurant and know you'll want one of their scrumptious desserts, don't deprive yourself or feel guilty if you eat it. Instead, consider choosing a lower calorie main dish at dinner or lunch. Or, you may decide to forego a drink at dinner because you know it is loaded with calories and you'd prefer the dessert. If you don't adjust your eating that day, consider increasing your exercise a bit the next day. No matter what you do, that cake will not be the end of the world. If you decide to eat it, make your choice about what you are going to do to balance your intake, and then forget about it.

Take these food strategies with a grain of salt. Use what you want. Use them as a resource or skip through them. You have to be in charge to make healthful choices. If a diet has control, you lose—no matter what it is called.

Personalize Your Strategy

As you review the food strategies, remember that each person is different. A food suggested in one plan may be a food that triggers a binge reaction to you. For instance, popcorn is very safe for some people and is helpful for avoiding a hypoglycemic reaction. For others, the smell of popcorn can trigger a binge. The most important aspect of selecting a food strategy is to use the least restrictive approach to food first. Using the Food and Feelings Monitor Chart in chapter 4 will help you identify foods that currently trigger you. It is certainly strategically wise to avoid those foods initially. After some time, you may choose to reintroduce them—one at a time. Make sure you reintroduce foods when you feel very safe and secure in your life and when the reintroduction is a choice—not a need.

Frequently, food strategies recommend avoiding sugar. Many people with weight problems make that decision for a variety of reasons, including hypoglycemia and allergies. Others may be able to maintain some sugar in their diets. For others, restricting sugar is a sure trigger to self-sabotage. It would not work. Don't try to con yourself. It is a time to be rigorously honest because you are doing this for yourself.

For a period of time, commit to one strategy without changing it. You set the time boundary. Individuals within Overeaters Anonymous (OA) make personal choices on how to refrain from compulsive overeating or to maintain abstinence one day at a time. They are encouraged to have a plan of eating, based on their individual needs. Many in OA find it extremely helpful to obtain what is called a food sponsor and read that person a list of the food scheduled for eating that day—committing their food one day at a time because looking at a lifetime of changed eating can be overwhelming. For some, this method would seem overly restrictive and not work at all. Others may find comfort in the structure. This method is not a requirement, but a choice. Whatever you choose, you will find the support within the OA meetings is helpful, too. The program is patterned after Alcoholics Anonymous and has meetings all over the United States and in sixty countries. In the United States, you can usually find OA listed in the telephone book.

The value of a plan of eating is that it helps serve as a guide. Some people benefit from the abstinence plans described; others' food strategy may include eating a certain number of meals a day.

Both can make life simpler. Either way, your personal commitment makes it more difficult to blame the diet as being restrictive and, therefore, to manipulate yourself out of control. Another way not to con yourself is to plan your meals ahead and, after eating, write them on the form provided in this book, at least for a few months. Planning not only gives you daily structure but also reduces the "need" to race to the shopping center when you are rushed and feeling depressed or overwhelmed. "Overwhelmed" often turns into "self-destruct." If you find yourself believing you are giving up everything for a food strategy, you will not stay on it long. It will be like a failed diet. It also may tap into some deep core feelings related to the fear of being deprived. Deprived of love. Deprived of attention.

If you begin to believe you are making new food choices as a tool to provide structure and stability in your life, you will feel less overwhelmed. You know you can lose weight. That's not really the issue. You probably have lost more weight and tried more diets than you like to remember. The key is to maintain some structure with your food and nourish your body and mind while you begin to nurture your soul with ongoing self-understanding and support. It also helps to think of this new way of eating as a nonrestrictive choice rather than as a diet. It may seem only a matter of semantics. However, diets are often associated with an obsessive need that has led to frequent failures and to corresponding low self-esteem.

Strategies for Hypoglycemia

Low blood sugar, or hypoglycemia, is often a problem for those with chronic weight issues, as well as for alcoholics and children of alcoholics. Oversecretion of insulin by the pancreas results in hypoglycemia, an abnormally low level of glucose (sugar) in the blood. Functional (or reactive) hypoglycemia has a direct relationship to the time and type of meal eaten. Hypoglycemics often have abnormal protein and carbohydrate metabolism. Stress can also trigger these types of hypoglycemic reactions.

Symptoms of Hypoglycemia

There is much controversy within the medical field about what magic number actually constitutes hypoglycemia. If, after you take a glucose tolerance test, your physician does not think you are hypoglycemic, yet you experience some of the following symptoms, you may still want to consider the hypoglycemic food strategy in this chapter. Learn to trust your body's own messages.

Identifying Symptoms of Hypoglycemia

Allergies
Anorexia
Anxiety
Blurred vision
Chronic indigestion
Cold hands or feet
Confusion
Craving for sweets
Crying spells
Depression
Dizziness
Dry or burning mouth
Emotional outbursts
Exhaustion
Fainting or blackouts
Headaches
Hot flashes
Impotence
Insomnia
Irritability when meals are missed

Irritability after eating a food
    that triggers an increase or
    decrease in blood sugar
Memory loss
Moodiness
Muscle pains, backache
Nervousness
Night sweats
Noise and light sensitivity
Obesity
PMS
Ravenous hunger between
    meals
Restlessness
Shakiness
Swollen feet
Tachycardia (palpitation of
    the heart)
Temper tantrums
Weakness

Physicians as Informed Partners

Many of these symptoms mimic other diseases. That is why it is imperative you have a physician as your partner in recovery. To promote evaluation for any other problems, advise your physician of all your symptoms when you request a glucose tolerance test. Remember, not all hypoglycemics crave sugar.

If you discover you are diabetic, you should carefully follow your doctor's advice about how to eat and about what to do when you have a hypoglycemic reaction. Hypoglycemia can be life-threatening.

Triggers of Hypoglycemia

Functional hypoglycemia, which is not accompanied by diabetes, is generally not life threatening—although it certainly can be regarded as life altering and can have serious consequences. If you reach for sugar to feel better or to satisfy a craving, you would achieve more stability if you opted for a protein food, a fiber food, and a glass of juice.

Sugar can cause an immediate change in feelings. Blood sugar may spike, then follow with a steep drop that often increases cravings for more sugar or alcohol—or makes the hypoglycemic more tired, grouchy, or severely ill. Those with hypoglycemia may awaken and feel as if they have hangovers—even though they have never ingested alcohol—or they may be extremely tired even after a full night's sleep. Because alcohol could be considered a liquid sugar, hypoglycemics should avoid it. When hypoglycemics eat something with sugar, they must be prepared for the possibility that food may have adverse effects, and they must carefully monitor their physical and emotional reactions. Many hypoglycemic food strategies recommend total abstinence from sugar and other products that can produce the same reaction. Other ingredients to look for in food labels include sucrose, glucose, maltose, dextrose, lactose, fructose, syrup, and honey. Notice that you will find many of these in so-called health or diet foods, in marinating sauce for meats, and on toppings for hams and some delicatessen meats.

However, you can make wise choices by monitoring your own reactions. You may be able to offset the sugar by increasing protein at the time you eat or drink. In that way you will not feel as if you are depriving yourself.

Most agree that those with functional hypoglycemia respond negatively to stress. It is essential, therefore, that you pay particular attention to maintaining healthful eating choices when life places a high level of stress upon you—even after you have been in recovery for the emotional causes. Do not overlook the impact of chronic stress upon your body, either. Those with depression or anxiety related to their weight tend to shoulder an enormous amount of job stress and need to set boundaries to protect themselves physically as well as emotionally.

Food Choices if You're Hypoglycemic

When to Eat? Hypoglycemics should eat six to eight meals a day to avoid blood sugar swings. You may find it helpful to eat every two to three hours. If you are not diabetic, eat a combination of high fiber with protein to stabilize a blood sugar swing. Combine crackers, bran with raw cheese or almond butter, or an apple. Fiber in popcorn, rice bran, and crackers slows reactions. A glass of fruit juice provides a rapid rise in blood sugar.

What to Eat? Some professionals recommend a low-carbohydrate diet combined with a daily intake of 11 ounces of protein from meat, fish, and poultry. However, others believe the need for protein is much lower—especially meat protein, which can contribute to some diseases. They recommend a diet of complex, high-quality carbohydrates (fruits, vegetables, and whole grains), high in fiber, and with less protein. Both diets avoid concentrated fruits, because they can create a sugar reaction within the body.

Many nutritionists recommend abstaining from refined foods such as instant rice and potatoes, white flour, soft drinks, alcohol, and salt, and avoiding sweet fruits and juices such as grape and prune juice (or diluting them with water). Your physician or nutritionist may be able to help you with a specific plan. The plan that follows gives you an idea of a possible structure for a day's needs if you're hypoglycemic.

Food Choices for Hypoglycemics

Protein: Up to 11 ounces. Cottage cheese may be included.

Fruit: 2 servings.

Vegetables: 2 to 4 servings.

Oil: Maximum 5 teaspoons (include what is used in cooking and on salads).

Milk: Skim or defatted buttermilk, 2 cups.

Bread: There is some debate about eating bread because the starch can create a sugar reaction. The key is learning to monitor your reactions. You may have up to 1/2 slice with meals and snacks without any problems. Or, you may want to substitute rice cakes or any of the following vegetables: a 1/2 cup beets, pumpkin, carrots, onions, peas, rutabagas, turnips, or winter squash. Again, remember that each person reacts differently to foods. Some have identified rice cakes as a binge food.

Food supplements may also be helpful. Consult a nutritionist or specialist to determine what may meet your needs. Many recommended supplements can be found in good multivitamins rich in B vitamins, and in amino acid supplements that provide protein. Some supplements and product claims include the following:

- **Chromium:** May help maintain blood sugar levels; important in the metabolism of glucose; found in brown rice, cheese, meat, dried beans, chicken, corn, calf's liver, and potatoes.
- **Niacin:** Important in the metabolism of carbohydrates, fats, and proteins. You may find that niacin produces a strong reaction, such as intense flushing. If that is a problem, try a timed-release capsule with meals and take an aspirin about 15 minutes prior to taking the supplement. Tolerance often increases with use. Niacin is in eggs, fish, tomatoes, carrots, and whole wheat.
- **Magnesium:** Important in calcium and potassium intake; in fish, meat, seafood, apples, bananas, brown rice, garlic, lima beans, nuts, black-eyed peas, green leafy vegetables, whole grains, and many other foods.
- **Vitamin B-12:** Also important in protein synthesis and metabolism of carbohydrates and fats. Available in tofu and from animal sources including eggs, kidney, mackerel, milk, seafood, and cheese.
- **Vitamin B complex:** Useful in energy production.
- **Spirulina:** Helps stabilize blood sugar between meals.
- **Vitamin C plus bioflavonoids:** Improves energy.
- **Zinc:** Essential for protein synthesis; in fish, meats, legumes, poultry, seafood, whole grains, egg yolks, liver, pecans, soybeans, and other foods.
- **L-Glutamine:** Amino acid reduces cravings for sugar.
- **L-Cysteine:** Amino acid blocks action of insulin.
- **Proteolytic enzymes:** Helps digest protein.
- **Manganese:** Essential for protein and fat metabolism. In blueberries, egg yolks, legumes, spinach, green leafy vegetables, and other foods.

Strategies for Coping with Food Allergies

If you experience discomfort after eating, you may have sensitivities or allergies to foods. Frequently, these are the very foods folks with weight problems crave or binge with. Some symptoms may indicate allergies; others may be red flags for different problems. Again, make a physician your partner in recovery. If possible, consult with an allergy specialist for specific food testing to help you determine what foods are unhealthful for you.

The following is a list of possible allergic reactions to food. Carefully observe your reactions after you eat a suspicious food. Use the Symptom Connection Chart in this chapter, and be sure to take it with you when you visit an allergy specialist. (Some chiropractors also strongly support their patients in discovering how food affects them and in suggesting allergy-free options and food supplements.)

Allergic Reactions

Acne	Constipation
Anger	Coughing
Anxiety	Cramps
Apathy	Dark circles under eyes
Asthma	Depression
Belching	Diarrhea
Bingeing on certain foods or drink	Dizziness
	Drowsiness
Blurred vision	Dry skin
Canker sores	Earache
Chest pain (Any time you feel chest pain, you must notify your physician as soon as possible.)	Excessive drooling
	Excessive sweating
	Feeling weak or tired
	Flushing
Chronic fatigue	Frequent or urgent urination
Compulsive eating	Gas
Confusion	Genital itch or discharge

Hair loss

Headaches

Heartburn

Hives

Hoarseness

Hyperactivity

Insomnia

Irregular heartbeat

Irritability

Lack of energy

Learning disabilities

Loss of voice

Low blood sugar

Memory problems

Mental dullness

Mood swings

Nausea

Need to clear your throat

Nervousness

Other illnesses

Pain in joints

Pain in muscles

Pain or sores in mouth or
     on lips

Poor coordination

Rashes

Repeated colds (in children)

Restlessness

Ringing in ears

Scratchy throat

Severe menstrual cycles

Shortness of breath

Sinus problems

Sluggishness

Sore throat

Sticky eyelids

Stiffness

Stomach pains

Stuffiness

Swollen eyes

Swollen tongue, gums, lips

Under- or overweight

Vomiting (associated only with
     a particular food. Bulimics
     are not purging due to
     allergies)

Water retention

Watery, itchy, red eyes

List other symptoms you may have.

1. _____

2. _____

3. _____

Food-Allergy Connection Chart

Copy the chart on page 160 and use it for two to four weeks to investigate whether there is a connection between your symptoms and particular foods, drinks, and medications.

When you have noted a reaction after a specific food, eliminate it from your diet for about two months. If you suspect an allergy or sensitivity to more than one food or drink, eliminate each one. By avoiding allergic foods and drinks for about two months, your body may have time to heal from the reaction. Then, you may test the food or drink you previously reacted to by reintroducing one food or drink at a time and carefully observing any reaction. If you connect an adverse reaction with a medication, contact your physician immediately. Your physician may be able to suggest an alternative.

Make your environment as safe as possible. As you discover what foods trigger a reaction, you have a choice. Some people function best if they eliminate these foods totally from the house. Others say they prefer to keep them—out of immediate sight. Others stock an abundance of these foods in the pantry because they say just knowing they are there makes them less tempting. You want to avoid feeling deprived, because that can trigger your reaching for food that may not be healthful for you. However, easy access makes you more vulnerable to using that food instead of alternatives. Only you can honestly answer what is best for you.

When you make a decision, you are in control, not your allergy diet, a condition that reduces the potential for not maintaining healthy eating because you feel controlled and trapped. By deciding for yourself, you convert a diet to a strategy.

Hidden Surprises

After you have noticed a pattern to your reactions, you may not realize how many foods contain your allergen. Circle the products that you did not realize contained the following ingredients, all of which are common allergens:

Food/Drinks	Time Eaten	Medication	Time Taken	Symptom	Time Noticed

The following may contain **wheat**:

Beer (sugar, too)

Biscuits

Bologna

Cakes (sugar, too)

Chocolate candy (sugar, too)

Cooked meat dishes

Cookies

Crackers

Doughnuts

Dumplings

Flour

Gravy

Liverwurst

Lunch meat

Pasta

The following may contain **yeast**:

Alcohol (beer, wine and liquor)

Barbecue sauce (often high in sugar)

Breads

Cakes

Catsup

Cereals

Crackers

Enriched flour

Horseradish

Mayonnaise

Pickles

Pretzels

Salad dressing

Sauerkraut

Vinegar

Vitamins (most are available
yeast-free. Read the label.)

The following may contain **corn**:

Aspirin

Beer

Bleached flour

Bourbon

Candy

Catsup

Cheese

Chewing gum

Cured ham

Distilled vinegar

Frozen fruits and vegetables

Gravy

Grits

Ice cream

Instant tea

Jam, jelly

Margarine

Pie crusts

Popcorn

Powdered sugar

Sandwich spreads

Toothpaste

Tortillas

Vitamins (Read the label.)

The following may contain **egg**:

Baking powder	Icing
Bread	Meat loaf
Breaded food	Meringue
Cake	Noodles or pasta
Cake flour	Sauces
Frying batters	Salad dressing
Hamburger mix	Sherbet
Hollandaise sauce	Soufflés
Ice cream	Tartar sauce

The following may contain **monosodium glutamate (MSG)**:

Accent	Dry soup mix
Canned soup and vegetables	Mayonnaise
Chinese food (many restaurants will allow you to special order MSG-free foods)	Packaged meats
	Potato chips
	Soy sauce

The following foods may contain **cottonseed oil**:

Barbecue sauce	Pasta
Commercial bread and cake	Pies
Commercial popcorn	Potato chips
Cottonseed flour	Rolls
Lard	Rye bread
Margarine	Salad dressing
Matzo	Sardines in oil

The following may contain **milk**:

Bread	Custard
Cake	Fritters
Cocoa drinks	Mashed potatoes
Cookies	Pie crusts
Crackers	Scalloped dishes
Creamed foods	

The following may contain **soy** or **soy oil**:

Asian sauces	Margarine
Baby food	Milk substitutes
Butter substitutes	Pork link sausage
Cake oil	Salad dressing
Ice cream	Soybean noodles
Lecithin	Soy flour
Lunch meat	Tofu

The following may contain **sulfites**:

Avocado (guacamole) dip	Horseradish
Baked products (frozen dough)	Lettuce
Beer	Lobster
Carrots	Mushrooms
Cider	(canned or fresh)
Clams	Onion relish
Cole slaw	Oyster
Corn, maple, and pancake syrups	Peppers
Crab	Pickles
Dried fish	Potatoes
French fries (frozen)	Potato chips
Fresh shellfish	Salad dressing (dry mixes)
Fruit	Sauerkraut
Fruit juice	Scallops
Fruits and vegetables	Shrimp
(frozen, canned, or dried)	Soup
Gelatin	Tomatoes
Grapes	Wine

The following may contain **sugar**:

Canned vegetables (Read the labels.)	Fast food
Catsup	French fries
Chinese food	Natural breakfast cereals

| Desserts | Peanut butter |
| Diet ice cream | Salad dressing |

Be cautious if you are triggered by sugar. Sugar and salt are often the top ingredients in canned foods. Many low-calorie offerings contain sugar. You may discover a surprising world when you begin to screen the ingredient list on foods you buy. Always read the ingredient list. Many people can safely have sugar if it is the fifth ingredient or lower.

Detox Is Not Unusual
As your body stops reacting to and starts eliminating the toxicity from certain foods, it is common to experience detoxification symptoms. These withdrawal symptoms can be very uncomfortable for up to two weeks. You may feel tired and irritable, and you may crave the foods you have discovered are the most dangerous for you. You may feel a ravenous hunger, and your body may ache. Although these symptoms are uncomfortable, your body's reaction should present a clear message to you regarding the effect those foods were having on your body. At about two weeks, most people report feeling more energy and less anxiety.

You may find that a particular food that you really enjoy is on your allergy list. Unless you can easily identify a payoff in not eating it, you may find it difficult to let go. There's a danger to you emotionally if you look at a food and think resentfully, "I can't eat that," instead of looking at a food and thinking "I don't want that because I'm choosing not to put up with its side effects." The "I can't" thinking is more likely to push you into feeling deprived or angry. While that combination of thinking and feeling may not lead you directly into eating the allergy food, it can pull you toward other dysfunctional eating. Eliminate the problem by acknowledging you are taking charge. Focus mentally on what you gain by refraining from eating those foods. These gains may include feeling less irritated, having more energy, and getting more sleep. Prepare for those moments in advance by writing your gains here.

Exercise: What I Have Gained by Avoiding Harmful Foods

1. _____

2. _____

3. _____

Always be rigorously honest in identifying all your feelings. Remember, feelings serve as messengers. Now note on the list below what you believe you have given up. In this way, you can compare the lists to determine what is most important for you to improve your quality of life. Is choosing to eliminate a food worth what you gain? Do you choose to reduce its use or eliminate it completely? This process also helps you recognize that what you are doing is a choice, not an obligation. Write the losses. Then compare them with your gains.

What I Have Lost by Giving Up This Food

1. _____

2. _____

3. _____

Food Sensitivities List

Because you have spent some time discovering the connection between specific foods and how you feel, it will be helpful for you to maintain a list of sensitive foods for future reference. Ironically, the healthier you become, the more you will recognize a reaction from eating food or drinking beverages that you are sensitive to. If you view this list as another essential life recovery tool, you will gradually memorize the list of foods that may harm you. Begin your list here, and make a copy for your kitchen, wallet, or purse.

Food Sensitivity List

Dairy products: _____

Vegetables: _____

Fruit: _____

Meat: _____

Grains or nuts: _____

Additive substances: _____

Herbs, seasonings: _____

Sweeteners:_____

Caffeine: _____

Sugar products: _____

Rotation Food Strategy

Many nutritionists recommend that people with allergies rotate their foods on four-day cycles, with no food eaten more often than every four days. By alternating foods, you reduce the risk of continuously eating a food that may trigger a reaction. You may then choose to eliminate the food completely, if you discover sensitivity.

Select your meals from an accepted food strategy, such as one recommended by the American Heart Association. Or, perhaps your doctor or nutritionist has one that includes all the basic food groups and provides a good selection to choose from. Most people find it is helpful to use a form to monitor and plan their rotation meals. Use the form on page 167 to plan your meal choices:

Among the numerous weight loss programs, the Weight Watchers plan is probably one of the most healthful. Over the years, it has added increased freedom of choice. This plan can be used in conjunction with your other important emotional work. However, remember to avoid obsessive focus and emotional rewards based on what the scales show.

Rotation Strategies				
Meal	Day 1	Day 2	Day 3	Day 4
Breakfast				
Lunch				
Dinner				
Snacks				

Eating for Perfection: Abstinence

Some professionals recommend that you rigidly adhere to a total abstinent food strategy, such as the one that follows. The benefit is that it takes all the questions out of eating. Amounts of and allowed foods are spelled out carefully. The danger is that you may become obsessed with perfection. Total abstinence lacks many choices. Many people relapse into depression after a period of abstinence because they have not worked through deep issues related to the use of food. All their energy has been focused on being "good" and maintaining total abstinence. When these intense feelings are triggered, the desire to use food can become overwhelming. Others believe in the benefits of abstinence so strongly that they swear total abstinence has saved their lives and is necessary for its continuation.

The most important aspect of your food choice is that it be put in perspective. Structure can be effective in providing a safety net during a time when you may feel out of control.

Many people use intensely structured abstinent food strategies, especially people who consider themselves to be food addicts. If you engage in this highly structured approach, find sponsors in support groups. They can be very helpful, especially if you have questions concerning food choices. Be aware though: Many people adhere to the structure rigidly and may not accept any flexibility. They may also discount the importance of therapy and self-discovery. Others, however, have adopted a holistic approach to recovery. Listen and observe as you select your support system. Those who choose an abstinence plan often will also use a twelve-step approach, similar to Overeaters Anonymous and Alcoholics Anonymous. They regard veering from abstinent eating as slips. Participants are encouraged to learn from the experience and then to return to abstinent eating.

Abstinent Food Strategy

The abstinent food strategy requires total abstinence from any food not listed, although the list can vary. Within this food plan, certain foods are identified as trigger foods. Foods that contain flour, such as bread and pasta, are cited as common binge foods. Foods that are sweet and smooth or salty and crunchy are common trigger foods. In other words, people react to the texture of foods, which may trigger a binge response even though the food may be included in the list of foods that are okay to eat in an abstinent food strategy. Examples of trigger foods include popcorn and rice cakes as crunchies, peanut butter and cream cheese as smoothies.

In this plan, the goal is to eat food in its most whole, unrefined form, which tends to decrease exposure to texture and trigger foods. The plan does not include bacon, sausage, and deep-fried foods. It is high in fiber. Proponents believe this decreases the risk of heart disease and cancer, stabilizes blood sugar levels, helps promote satiety, and reduces cravings. Sometimes people beginning this food plan will have gas and stomach problems because of its high fiber content. These problems should dissipate within a short time, but if not, consult a physician.

This plan includes specific food measurements. Those who strictly adhere to the plan use scales to measure amounts. This measuring has been particularly helpful to anorexics who tend to cheat on amounts and to those who have overeaten based on years of medicating their feelings with foods. Those who find benefit with this plan find it reassuring and helpful. However, you may find it embarrassing to weigh and measure food in restaurants.

The plan calls for fish or chicken at least once a day. Beef, pork, and veal are limited to three times per week. Do not repeat any starchy vegetable or grain more than three times per week. Soy protein, such as tofu, can be used as a protein substitute at least once per week. Avoid eating one food all the time, or it may become a binge food. The plan usually includes using multivitamins.

On this plan, most people who are overweight can lose a substantial amount of weight in a year. Anorexics may be overwhelmed with the amount of food in this plan; some have successfully used a version of this plan by starting with smaller amounts of the foods required. They tend to gain some weight, but not a large amount. The gain may seem unreasonable to them, but a health official may contend that the food plan will help them maintain weight within a healthy range.

Many people consult with nutritionists after about six months on the plan to determine if any adjustments need to be made. They are then placed on a maintenance plan. This abstinent strategy is designed for adults but has been used with all age groups. Consult your nutritionist or doctor for changes based on age or for questions about any health issues.

Whatever food strategy you choose, it is also of prime importance that you eat on time. The plan encourages you to use relaxed eating and forces you to take time out for meals. This scheduling is important whether or not you choose to follow a specific plan. The technique of putting your fork down between bites slows emotional eating and weight gain. The abstinent food strategy encourages those using vegetarian proteins to combine them with meat or cheese. Participants are encouraged to limit salt intake and use a wide variety of herbs and spices.

Abstinence Choices

For Females:

Breakfast	Lunch	Dinner
1 fruit	1 c. vegetables	1 c. vegetables
1 cereal	3 oz. protein	3 oz. protein
8 oz. skim milk	1/2 c. starch	1/2 c. starch
1 protein	1 c. salad	1 c. salad
	1 fat	1 fat
	1 fruit	clear broth (optional)

Snack
1 fruit
1 cereal
8 oz. skim milk

For Males:

Breakfast	Lunch	Dinner
1 fruit	1 fruit	
1 cereal	1 fat	1 fat
1 protein	4 oz. protein	4 oz. protein
8 oz. skim milk	1 c. salad	1 c. salad
	1/2 c. starch	1 c. starch
	1 c. vegetables	1 c. vegetables
	clear broth	

Snack
1 fruit
1 cereal
8 oz. skim milk

Fruits: 1 whole, 1 cup fresh, 1/2 cup canned or 1 cup frozen (thawed). Fresh fruit, 1 cup allowance: apples, apricots, blackberries, blueberries, boysenberries, cantaloupe (melon, honeydew), cranberries, lemons or limes (3 small), oranges, pears, pineapple, raspberries, rhubarb tangerines, or watermelon. No cherries, grapes, kiwi fruit, mango, or papaya. The following are exceptions: 2 medium bananas (no more than twice a week), 1/2 grapefruit, 2 small nectarines, peaches, or plums.

Condiments: 1/2 cup allowance per meal. Barbecue sauce, horseradish, mustard, salsa (be aware of sugar content), soy sauce, all spices, and Worcestershire sauce. Steak sauce, horseradish, and mustard are not to exceed 1 tablespoon per meal.

Vegetables: 1 cup allowance. Alfalfa sprouts, asparagus, bean sprouts, beans (green, wax, Italian), bok choy, beets, broccoli*, Brussels sprouts, cabbage, carrots, cauliflower, celery, chard, collard, cucumbers, dandelion greens*, eggplant, lettuce, mushrooms, mustard, okra, onions, turnip, parsley, peppers (bell, red, green, chili, jalapeno), pickles (dill), radishes, rutabagas, sauerkraut, snow peas, summer squash, spinach*, tomatoes, turnips, water chestnuts, yellow turnips, zucchini. *Limit to one serving per day because of high vitamin A content.

Proteins: 3 oz. for women, 4 oz. for men each day. Cooked with excess fat removed before weighing. All lean beef, all lean lamb, all lean pork (excluding bacon and sausage, which are high in fat and sodium), all lean veal, all lean shellfish, chicken (breast, thigh, or leg), plain tuna. Cold protein should be selected no more than 3 times a week. Cottage cheese, farmer cheese, feta cheese, pot cheese, ricotta cheese. No hard cheese until maintenance is agreed upon with nutritionist.

Breakfast protein choices include 1/4 cup ricotta cheese or cottage cheese, 1/2 cup plain lowfat or nonfat yogurt, 2 oz. or 1 egg soft or hardboiled or scrambled in a nonstick skillet.

Beverages: Any sugar-free, decaffeinated beverage, decaf coffee, tea, limited to 4 cups daily. Decaf sugar-free soda limited to 2 per day. **Drink 8 to 10 8-ounce glasses of water per day.**

Salad: Measure carefully: 1 cup for lunch and 1 cup for dinner.

Fat: 1 teaspoon oil, margarine, butter, or mayonnaise at lunch and 1 teaspoon at dinner. You may substitute a commercial dressing in which 1 tablespoon will be equivalent to 1-teaspoon oil or margarine.

Starchy Vegetables: 1/2 cup at lunch and 1/2 cup at dinner. Corn, acorn squash, potatoes, peas, lima beans, kidney beans, 1/2 ear of corn, butternut squash, brown rice, wild rice, spaghetti squash, garbanzo beans (chickpeas), navy beans, barley, all dried beans, peas, lentils. Potatoes: baked small, boiled. Weight 4 oz., mashed, 1/2 cup.

Grains: 1 oz. dry measure for breakfast and 1 oz. for metabolic adjustment. Oat bran, Uncle Sam's cereal, shredded wheat, oatmeal, Grape-Nuts, puffed rice, wheat, or barley, and other cereals available at health food stores.

Other: Sweet 'n Low or Equal, no more than 6 servings per day. (This should be monitored in any food strategy. Some people substitute breath mints and candies with sweetener for sugar binges.) Lemon wedges, no more than 2 per meal; cinnamon, no more than 1/2 teaspoon per meal; vanilla, no more than 1 teaspoon per meal; sugar-free gum, no more than 6 pieces per day.

There are similar abstinence strategies that slightly change the amount or types of food allowed, yet remain based on following a highly structured plan.

The Exchange Plan

The American Dietetic Association offers an exchange plan as another alternative. In coordination with a registered dietitian, you put together a program with specific guidelines on carbohydrates, starches, fruit, milk, meat, and fat for each meal. In each category, you are provided lists of foods that you may exchange. This flexibility prevents you from becoming bored and gives you freedom of choice.

Recovery Checklist

As you change your eating habits, chart your recovery. This is another method to help you validate your success and not let the scales continue to tell you how to feel. Review your checklist frequently, and use it daily or weekly for three months. Here is an example:

1. I feel more energy.
2. I notice less irritability around mealtime.
3. I feel less confused.
4. I am sick less frequently.
5. I have fewer physical pains.
6. _____
7. _____

Dangers of Food Strategies

The danger with any food strategy is that it can become an obsession. Adherence to the strategy can be used much the same way food is used: as a means to dissociate from problems. It is dangerous to trade an obsession with weight, bingeing, or purging with a perfectionist attitude toward eating. Thus, veering from your strategy (as any human being eventually will) becomes a means to sabotage recovery. Any slip from perfect eating can perpetuate the shame of not being able to do anything right. It also can feed into deep feelings related to being deprived, as mentioned previously. *The people who do best with a food strategy over the long term are those who regard it as a choice that helps them feel good*, not those who think that with almost every bite they will never be able to eat "normally" again.

Never allow someone else to shame you, either. If you veer from the food strategy for a meal, for a day, or for a month, remember that all you have to do is get back on it during the next meal. Hopelessness or feelings of imperfection will only push you into a destructive cycle of overeating, not eating, bingeing, purging, or just giving up.

Throughout it all, remain rigorously honest. If you find you are using any strategy as a tool to sabotage yourself and provide an excuse to delve into old behaviors, you may want to reconsider your approach to food selection.

Remember: It's Your Choice; It's Your Life

Each person is different. Decisions about your food and your future should be made from a base of your knowledge and your beliefs. Give yourself time to discover what kind of eating pattern is best for you. Self-persecution sometimes occurs when you do not follow your own strategic choices. Very quickly, it can feel like another failed diet. However, there is one major difference. This time you have information. You know that one more diet is not the answer. No magic diet will make your life change. The change must come from within. It takes learning how to nurture yourself. It takes education. It takes knowledge of how emotions affect your eating and an honest look at society's unrealistic expectations concerning obtaining the perfect weight.

Never give away to food the power of your life or your recovery. Believe in your ability to make choices. You have worked hard to identify and decrease the interference of issues other than hunger affecting what you eat. In the last chapter, we're going to take a look at how far you have come and of what will continue to sustain your experience. We'll also celebrate hope, the emotion that pulled you into this journey and that will sustain you through the most difficult times.

AFFIrmation
Today I rejoice in my own growth
and acknowledge
I have the ability to make independent choices.

---| **11** |---

CELEBrate your Transformation

Hope is the anchor of the soul, the stimulus
to action, and the incentive to achievement.

—Anonymous

Years of frustration trying to lose weight can rob you of hope, one of life's most powerful gifts. Yet, it was hope, a small flame that burns despite whatever we have been through, that pulled you into this journey. Hope, partnered with what you have learned, will continue to blossom as new opportunities become open to you.

When Karen began working the same steps you have, she expressed disbelief that life could ever change. She was suffering from depression as a result of childhood incest and had struggled with out-of-control eating for years. However, a remnant of hope, coupled with her willingness to work, allowed her to progress through the same steps you have, one at a time, and to make changes in her life that far surpassed her initial concerns about her physical appearance. Her struggles in self-discovery have been intense, yet healing. She said, "Never in my life would I have imagined I could feel this wonderful and as calm and peaceful inside. As I read and completed the exercises, little by little my hope increased. As I worked, I also developed a relationship with God and I found strength. Even though there are a lot of chaotic things in my life, I have this calmness inside I have never had before. That negative chatterbox is gone. I know how to stop it.

"I believe there is a future for me now. I believe I am loveable. People love me, find me attractive, and care about me—the person. I love myself and never before in my life could I ever have said those words. Sometimes I love myself so much I am my best friend. God loves me. It just feels so wonderful to be able to say those things. I am a capable person."

Today, you and Karen do not have to doubt that capability, even when the scales fluctuate. You can look in the mirror with acceptance for the person you are and recognize that you have much to offer the world. If you have a difficult day and self-doubt begins to creep in, or if you find yourself again focusing on outward appearance, you have the knowledge to step back and access what is going on in your life right now. Drawing from the information you have gathered, you will be able to address problems before they get out of control and not revert back to destructive coping mechanisms or that negative chatterbox that Karen refers to.

"When you release all those old uncomfortable feelings," Karen added, "you get through to that other side and let go of a past. I have a life where not every thought is of pain, and I don't obsess over what I weigh."

Karen's journey, while inspiring, is not unusual for those who work through these steps of change. Like all of us, she always had amazing potential within. Given some focused direction, gentle nurturing, and more effective tools, she became like the butterfly set free of a cocoon. Today she faces the world unencumbered by past pain, distorted perceptions, and overwhelming negative thoughts about herself. She has a job she only dreamed of and a husband who loves her for who she is inside. The scales no longer tell her who she is. Karen tells the world who she is. Look out!

Step 10: Review your progress, take note of your changes and celebrate yourself!

By this time, that transition has also started occurring within you. The changes may seem small, but remember these serve as the catalyst to powerful transitions. As you've seen, small changes provide strong building blocks to help you successfully tackle problems in all aspects of life. It is important that you celebrate each of these changes. While they may seem inconsequential to some, you know how significant each has been to your progress. Celebrating these changes has been important for Karen, just as it is for you.

You know how significant it is to be able to say no to people, to set boundaries with people you love, and not to fall into old behavior. While it may seem insignificant to someone else that you declined being a chaperone on your child's field trip, recognize that not too long ago that action may have propelled you into guilt, anxiety, and knuckling under, even though you had no time.

Even though these processes will not be as difficult the more you practice, keep thinking that's big stuff. We too often neglect to congratulate ourselves along the way. Those congratulations and self-encouragement, in fact, continue to be the building blocks to sustaining a healthy emotional life.

Say Goodbye to Old Restraints

Recognition comes after a period of hard work, emotional sweat and self-understanding. You have begun to absorb what you have learned and to replace old negative thoughts about yourself with new core beliefs. You are no longer restricted by unclaimed emotions and a misguided focus on your weight. Most people describe these changes as freedom.

Think about what new freedoms you have achieved and about the potential you have as your confidence about who you are becomes commonplace. Like you, Karen knew she had made a big step in her life when she was able to tell someone no without having to focus all her attention just on getting the words out, then fighting back guilt. Previously, she would do what she did not want to do, feel used and resentful, and then turn to food to take those feelings away. Today, she is able to devote energy to activities that she finds satisfying and joyful, instead of giving all of herself to others who are not appreciative or supportive. She is able to revert to the tools she has learned in order to keep herself out of abusive relationships with friends, co-workers, men, and even food. When Karen started this adventure, she had no idea that her weight and image were so strongly tied to every other part of her life. Karen said, "I can look back in my journals and see how unhappy I was, how incapable I felt. I read my journals today and I am not the same person. It doesn't mean I was a bad person. I just didn't know how to take care of myself before. It's never too late. I'm thirty-four years old, and I feel as if I have just been born."

Discovering Yourself
You have entered this same process with your own unique history, but you have also discovered that you share many of the same experiences, feelings, and thoughts of Karen and others who have struggled with their weight. Your journey has taken you into nooks and crannies you probably did not know existed, as you have worked to identify and let go of the accumulation of years of discouragement, brought upon by others and by yourself. As you've found, it hasn't always been easy. Delving into your relationships with your family has been tougher than the most stringent diet. Yet, through the process, you have learned new ways to express and care for yourself. You may discover as you continue to set your own identity that your family relationships will actually become more meaningful.

Karen encountered some rough spots from family members who preferred not to acknowledge the incest. Even today, she occasionally interprets their words as disapproving. She has learned, as you have, that while she cannot control their actions, she can control her reactions. She no longer absorbs their feelings but confronts her reactions by using the tools you have learned—grounding techniques, reality checks, and various techniques of expressing herself. In the past, she would have tried to ignore those feelings by using food. Karen has had some very positive results from establishing herself as an independent person within her family system. She no longer has to pretend to be who her parents or siblings want her to be, and she can be true to herself. In her unflinching honesty, she has found from others increased support and respect that she did not know she had. As a result of the changes Karen's mother saw in Karen, her mother has sought help for herself.

Karen continued, "It just seems so intense now because for the first time in years I am allowing myself to feel feelings without numbing out. In doing so, I am exorcising myself of a lot of guilt which I have learned I did not deserve. I am setting boundaries and I'm proud of them. Oh, sometimes I know I go back a little. But now I know how to refocus."

Karen knows she is stronger. Regarding her new strength, she said, "Even when I am afraid, I'm not bingeing, and what is surprising today is I don't even want to. I'm not driven to use the food anymore. Everything is coming together."

Feelings Set You Free

Connecting with feelings has been an essential part of your progress, as well. Today you are more tuned into listening to a feeling and to examining exactly what it signifies to you. This lights your path to determine what action is needed. You have learned to sift through past emotional trauma, to be able to fully enjoy the days you are living in now. Acknowledging the effects of loss has been difficult, because with that you have had to own the depth of your pain. Through your work, you have learned the importance of acknowledging the emotional consequences of that loss. Today, you are able to shed the tears and move forward, never forgetting the loss but no longer tied to it.

You are taking steps to maintain the powerful system of self-care that operates when you connect your head with your heart and body as a whole, carefully listening to and integrating the messages from each part of you. Letting go of this emotional pain is more difficult than changing the behaviors seen by the outside world. Today you don't have to jump into new diets to prove to the world that you agree with its assessment that your weight is a problem. Although you may still struggle with your weight at times, overall you know you are more than your weight. The knowing shows the growth you have achieved.

Looking Forward to Tomorrow

Unlike during your previous attempts to lose weight, you'll find you have experienced a lifestyle change. You'll want to continue to allow yourself to grow and venture into new territories. Explore whatever it is that you have always wanted to do but may not have had the confidence to do. As you go through difficult times in your life, pick up this book again. You will be surprised at how you relate, on a different level, to the same information as you continue to gain strength in your identity. Karen commented about her change within, "I am learning to look at life in awe and wonderment. I am learning to go out to eat and just enjoy the company of a friend. I do not have to be conscious of everything I put into my mouth. I do not have to wonder if everyone in the room is looking at me when I leave the table to go to the bathroom. Now I say, 'What of it?' If I believe someone is looking at me, I smile. I think it's because they sense in me a change. They want what I have.

"It is not something you buy off a rack or you gain when you lose twenty or thirty pounds. It is something you give yourself. A new patience with yourself allows you to explore who you are. To respect who you are. To finally feel I am good enough."

As you continue to practice new techniques and change old negative beliefs, you will feel more energy, power, and confidence. Like Karen, you will find yourself taking more risks and time to meet your dreams, instead of losing yourself in others. Hope, which may have been only a small spark inside or almost forgotten, kindles anew as you gain confidence from your work. You are making things happen in your life. As you continue, concerns about weight will drift away. No more frenzied dieting, giving up holiday festivities, or staying home alone trapped by a limited vision of who you are. Today, you don't need to look in the mirror to know who you are. There is a sense of greater acceptance, of knowing that eating a favorite food does not make you a bad person. Food and weight no longer define you. You're in charge. What a wonderful feeling! Absorb it! Live it!

AFFIRMATION:

Today I will celebrate myself as a whole person
who listens to and integrates the messages
of my head, heart, and body.

aPPenDIX

SIGnS anD SYMPTOMS
OF EaTInG DISOrDers

You have learned that difficulties with food can progress into eating disorders. The outlook for you to recover from these is very good. The information and techniques you've used throughout the book have served as effective tools for hundreds of people with eating disorders to move into recovery.

As you complete the following questionnaires, consider yourself on a fact-finding mission. There's nothing to be ashamed about if you have an eating disorder. If you find yourself answering yes to a number of these questions, you'll want to take your completed questionnaire with you and consult a physician and counselor for additional assistance. You're on your way to better health!

Anorexia

Anorexia is a progressive disease if untreated. If you recognize your own thoughts or behaviors in reading the definition and symptoms, you can find help to stop them and live an enriching life. If you have anorexia, you believe you are fat and have an intense fear of gaining weight or becoming fat, even if you are underweight; you refuse to have your weight at or above a minimally normal weight for your age and height. Circle the questions that reflect your behaviors or thoughts.

1. Are you a perfectionist?
2. Do other people comment about your being too thin?

3. Do you have a preoccupation with food? Do you find yourself planning meals for the family, doing the shopping, and then frequently not eating?

4. Do you appear calm on the surface but actually suffer from low self-esteem?

5. Do you rarely sit down or remain still?

6. Do you have a fear that others will be thinner?

7. Have you lost a significant amount of weight?

8. Have you ever lost weight to weigh what you believed would be acceptable and then discovered you needed to lose more?

9. Are you an overachiever?

10. Do you find yourself frequently not completing projects?

11. Do you have dry, flaking skin?

12. If you are a woman, have you stopped menstruating?

13. Do you frequently dress in sweaters, long-sleeve shirts, and other clothes to hide a thin appearance from family and friends?

14. Do you notice a heightened sensory experience, particularly sight, hearing, and sense of time?

15. Have you had a growth of fine body hair or lanugo?

16. Do you feel your intelligence, personality, or appearance is inferior?

17. Have you suffered a loss as a result of death, sexual abuse, divorce, or other life events?

18. Are you obsessed with exercise, fat, or calories?

19. Do you have obsessive-compulsive rituals? (These may include self-imposed rules on when you eat, how you eat, or where you will eat.)

20. Do you find yourself playing with food to make other people believe you are eating it?

21. Do you find yourself trying to meet the expectation of being the best little boy or girl in the world?

22. Do you have a lowered pulse rate?

23. Do you find yourself getting cold more frequently than those around you?

24. Do you have a fear of becoming obese that does not diminish as weight loss progresses?
25. Do you refuse to eat normally or at all?
26. Do you have periods when you don't eat a meal or avoid eating for more than a day?
27. Do you suffer from constipation?
28. Do you frequently feel depressed or hopeless?
29. Do you have a pattern of destructive relationships?
30. Do you have family, work, or money problems?

Bulimia

Since many people alternate from one eating disorder behavior to another, consider also if you are exhibiting any signs of bulimia. Bulimia occurs after a period of binge eating, which is eating a larger amount of food than most people would eat in a short period of time or feeling a lack of control over what or how much you are eating. If you are bulimic, you work to prevent weight gain by using self-induced vomiting; taking a large number of laxatives, diuretics, or enemas; fasting; or excessive exercise. If you have bulimia, your perception of your body and weight is distorted and interferes with your life. In addition to the symptoms listed under Compulsive Overeating in chapter 2, purging bulimics frequently answer yes to the following questions. Circle those that apply.

1. Do you purchase and consume what you consider to be an enormous amount of food? (The amount varies with the individual. A cup may be a binge to one person; the inability to stop eating large quantities of food may be a binge to another.)
2. Do you believe that if you improve your body appearance it will improve your relationships?
3. Do you often think about a binge?
4. Did you learn to binge and purge as a means to control your weight?
5. Do you purge to relieve indigestion?

6. Have you used excessive laxatives or diuretics?

7. Are you often depressed?

8. Do you have puffiness in your face?

9. Do you feel out of control?

10. Do you ever vomit when you are not physically sick?

11. Are you recovering from chemical dependency?

12. Are you a child of a chemically dependent parent?

13. Have you ever used drugs to control eating?

14. Have you ever had physical symptoms such as weakness or dehydration?

15. Are you sensitive to rejection and connect rejection with your weight?

16. Do you depend upon others for your self-esteem?

17. Do you have secretive behavior?

18. Are you normal or slightly above what a physician would consider a healthy body weight?

19. Have you kept the bulimia a secret for some time?

20. Do you often feel hopeless?

21. If you are an adult, do you find your parents still dictating your life—even telling you how to feel?

22. Do you suffer from edema?

23. Do you have headaches?

24. Do you suffer from heart disease, diabetes, or arthritis?

25. Do you frequently feel guilty?

26. Are you a caretaker who spends more time helping others than helping yourself?

27. Did you switch roles while growing up, becoming the little father or little mother at a young age?

28. Have you learned to mask your true feelings?

29. Do you have poor impulse control?

30. Do you have problems in spending beyond your income?

31. Do you have excessive tooth decay or loss of tooth enamel?

32. Do you suffer from weakness or fatigue?

33. Do you have a chronic sore throat?
34. Do you have gastrointestinal disorders?
35. Do you frequently have physical problems?
36. Have you had periods when you lost total interest in sex or when you believed you were promiscuous?
37. Are you often irritable?
38. Do you believe no one really cares enough to understand you?
39. Do you find yourself trusting the wrong people?

If you recognize yourself from the definition and answered yes to a significant number of these questions, you need to tell your doctor you think you either have bulimia or are progressing toward that. Request lab tests, since bulimia can cause physical problems. Then congratulate yourself, because you have taken the hardest step in recovery. With your physician as your partner, you'll be able to use what you have learned in Body Sense as a strong base to continue in a long-term recovery.

Symptoms of Compulsive Exercising

Compulsive exercising, which is a form of bulimia, may include a combination of all the symptoms described. If you are a compulsive exerciser, you will use our society's emphasis on healthy exercise as a means to rationalize addictive behavior. Circle the questions that apply to you.

1. Do you feel driven to exercise?
2. Do you become upset if anything interferes with your exercise patterns?
3. Do you believe you must exercise more than one hour every day, regardless of any interruptions?
4. Would you rather exercise than be involved in a social interaction outside the exercise setting?
5. Do you minimize any physical pain that occurs as a result of exercising?
6. Do you lose yourself during exercise?

7. If you just completed an hour or two of strenuous exercise and a friend invites you to a movie, would you go?
8. If you just completed an hour or two of strenuous exercise and a friend invites you to jog or play tennis, would you go?
9. Do you isolate yourself?

If your answers were yes, consider that you may be bulimic. With help you can achieve a healthy balance in your life.

If you're concerned about your symptoms, see a doctor and enlist the help of a mental health counselor. You'll want one that will appreciate the work that you've done in *Body Sense*, and will help you delve more deeply into any troublesome areas where you need a little extra support.

As you can see, for many the battle with weight goes beyond dieting. If you have answered yes to a significant number of questions on any set, you owe it to yourself to gather more information. Explore further what maintains the destructive behavior and how to change. With help, you'll be feeling much better about yourself and how you look. Soon weight will no longer be your primary concern, freeing you to focus your energy on enjoying life and enhancing your relationships.

additional resources

I hope that your reading *Body Sense* will have reinforced your desire to keep learning and enriching your life. The following listings can help you in that ongoing endeavor. Just remember, Web addresses sometimes change. If you discover one that is not active, you may still be able to reach the organization by using a search engine.

Forgetaboutdiets.com and Recoverypaths.com
This Web site, coordinated by the author of Body Sense, *will provide you with ongoing support and information regarding many topics, including weight issues, relationships, trauma, depression, anxiety, and parenting. It also contains links to some of the latest research and current topics, as well as opportunities to ask the author questions online. It's a good place to receive ongoing support for the progress you've made. You can access it via either Web address.*

American Dietetic Association
This national organization provides nutritional tips and explanations.
216 Jackson Blvd.
Chicago, IL 60606
www.eatright.com

American Heart Association
You can find the Association's recommended healthful diet here.
American Heart Association National Center
7272 Greenville Ave.
Dallas, TX 75231
www.americanheart.org

Crisis Centers (local)

You can always call 911 or your local emergency number if you have a crisis. Those contacts are also available online:
www.befrienders.org/talk.htm

Cyberdiet.com

This site provides primarily diet and nutritional information, but it also looks at healthful versus dangerous diets. It has numerous online chat rooms available.

Doctors Who's Who

This online support site provides a wealth of information not only on eating disorders but on other health issues.
www.doctorswhoswho.com

Eating Disorders Awareness and Prevention (EDAP)

This is a national organization dedicated to increasing awareness of and preventing eating disorders. They provide educational materials and will answer questions.
www.edap.org

National Association to Advance Fat Acceptance (NAAFA)

This is an advocacy group promoting fat acceptance and fighting discrimination because of weight.
P.O. Box 188620
Sacramento, CA 95818

National Association of Anorexia Nervosa and Associated Disorders (ANAD)

Provides consumer advocacy, counseling referrals, and 24-hour hotline counseling at 847-831-3438.
P.O. Box 7
Highland Park, IL 60035
www.anad.org

National Institutes of Health

Provides summaries of research and health initiatives on treatment of obesity.

www.nhlbi.com

Oprah.com

This site has several supportive chat groups, and it features fitness training advice from Bob Greene, who co-authored the weight and fitness training book Make the Connection *with Oprah Winfrey. Their book has an especially good description of how to determine if you are operating at the optimal aerobic level.*

www.oprah.com

Overeaters Anonymous (OA)

This twelve-step organization is a fellowship of individuals who share their experiences, strength, and hope with the goal of abstaining from compulsive overeating. They have meetings all over the world. Their site provides information and non-judgmental support.

www.overeatersanonymous.org

Overeaters Anonymous World Service Office

6075 Zenith Court NE

Rio Rancho, NM 87124.

Somethingfishy.org

This is an excellent online information source on eating disorders, and it also includes chat rooms and online presentations.

BEYOND WORDS PUBLISHING, INC.

OUR CORPORATE MISSION:

Inspire to Integrity

OUR DECLARED VALUES:

We give to all of life as life has given us.

We honor all relationships.

Trust and stewardship are integral to fulfilling dreams.

Collaboration is essential to create miracles.

Creativity and aesthetics nourish the soul.

Unlimited thinking is fundamental.

Living your passion is vital.

Joy and humor open our hearts to growth.

It is important to remind ourselves of love.

To order or to request a catalog, contact:
Beyond Words Publishing, Inc.
20827 N.W. Cornell Road, Suite 500
Hillsboro, OR 97124-9808
503-531-8700 or 1-800-284-9673

You can also visit our Web site at *www.beyondword.com*
or e-mail us at *info@beyondword.com*.